HEALTH BY CHOCOLATE

radical new recipes & nutrition know-how

Victoria Laine

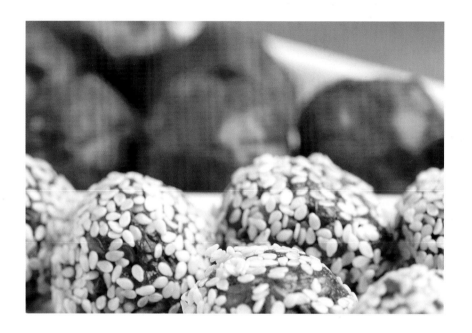

Foreword by John Robbins

OwL Medicine Books

Edmonton, Canada

HEALTH BY CHOCOLATE:
Radical New Recipes & Nutrition Know-How

Victoria Laine, with forewords by John Robbins and Sally Errey

OwL Medicine Books
PO Box 79042
926 Ash Street
Sherwood Park, AB
T8A 2G1

Copyright © 2008

Distributed by
Gordon Soules Book Publishers Ltd.
1359 Ambleside Lane,
West Vancouver, BC, Canada V7T 2Y9
E-mail: books@gordonsoules.com
Web site: http://www.gordonsoules.com
(604) 922 6588 Fax: (604) 688 5442

Every effort has been made to ensure that the information contained in this book is complete and accurate. However, neither the publisher nor the authors are engaged in rendering professional advice or services to the individual reader. The ideas, procedures, and suggestions contained in this book are not intended as a substitute for consulting a physician or health care professional. All matters regarding your health require responsible supervision.

The purpose of this book is to educate and entertain. Neither the author nor the publisher shall be liable or responsible for any loss, injury, or damage allegedly arising from any information or suggestion in this book.

It is recommended the recipes contained in this book be followed as written. The author and publisher are not responsible for your specific health or allergy needs that may require medical supervision. The author and publisher are not responsible for any adverse reactions to the recipes contained in this book.

If you do not wish to be bound by the above, you may return this book to the publisher for a full refund.

Recipes may be re-printed with written permission from the author. Re-prints must include credit to the author and book purchasing information. www.healthbychocolatebook.com -or- www.wholefoodsrescue.com (780) 416-4244.

Library and Archives Canada Cataloguing in Publication

Laine, Victoria, 1959-

Health by chocolate : radical new recipes & nutrition know-how / Victoria Laine ; foreword by John Robbins.

(Wholefoods to the rescue!)

Includes index.

ISBN 978-0-9784143-0-6

1. Cookery (Chocolate).   2. Chocolate--Health aspects.   I. Title.   II. Series.

QP144.C46L33 2007   641.6'374   C2007-905637-7

Edited by: Betty Putters

Design and Illustration: © David Shkolny

Photography: © Nanette Samol

Food Stylist: Victoria Laine and Nanette Samol

Printed in Canada by Friesens Printing

www.healthbychocolatebook.com

Thank you and Acknowledgements

I certainly didn't create this book alone, but I did lure each friend and family member involved, into my chocolate book obsession with my endless ideas and questioning. Thankfully, you all encouraged it! Thank you all for your patience and support of this book. The process of writing and compiling it has been a blessed gift to me, far reaching and healing than I could ever have imagined. The angels that arrived to assist the process was divine confirmation 'to go for it"!!

The HEALTH BY CHOCOLATE Team!

Wow, what good fortune and fun I've had working with the talented people that have come into my life for this book project!

David Shkolny, (B.F.A., Nova Scotia College of Art and Design) illustrator, graphic designer and educator, is also a talented artist whose work can be found in international collections. His creativity brought the book to life and his commitment to the project from the start has made him a pleasure to work with. I am grateful for your patience and generosity to my first book project David! Thank you. Contact **DAVID SHKOLNY DESIGN** at drawingteach@gmail.com

Nanette Samol, (B.A., Augustana University College, Dip. Photojournalism, Western Academy of Photography) is a doubly talented food stylist and photographer with a passion for excellence. Professional, with flexibility and commitment, she is sought after for her creativity and style. Thank you Nanette!

Glenda Wyatt, was the reason this book was completed. You came into my life years earlier as a yoga student, and offered one day to help me complete my book. Little did you know what you were getting into (nor did I!) You sacrificed and volunteered hours on the computer, inputting, organizing, giving constant feedback and keeping me on track, and as long as I fed you chocolate you were happy. Your support, without taking from my process, was wise and brilliant. I'm forever indebted my friend.

Betty Putters, thank you for your generous and careful editing…and in record time!

Jan, my 'younger' sister and supporter, is the other reason this book is complete. Your patience with endless (sleepless) hours - keeping me on track, washing dishes, editing, encouraging, listening and a gazillion other services you've provided is remarkable! You are appreciated more than you'll ever know.

Mariah and Jacqueline, my dear supportive daughters. Without a doubt there is a special place for you in the Abha' Kingdom, along with other children of authors! I am blessed and grateful in a way no words can express.

Cheering Team, Dishwashers, Recipes Testers and Tasters, Manuscript Readers and Editors and Other Essential Assistance – Mom, Dad, Jan, Sarah, Manizheh and Kevin, Shar and Redwan, Sonya and Paul, Hugh, Michele, Lorene and Mladin, Val and Peter, Tara, Deb, Peggy, Sheila, Adrienne, Fiona, Michel, Jeannne-Marie, Autumn, Angie, Cathy Anne, Mark and many other cherished friends. Thank you for all of your gracious encouragement, feedback and input, suggestions, dish loans and service. Thank you to **Sharzad** for the title idea. Thank you to **Frank** for the donation of a large mass of chocolate for the photo shoot. A special thank you to **Elke** for her magical massages, where the ideas flow like a river of chocolate! I'm forever grateful to you all!

To the **Campbell family** for helping me kickstart my career.

And last, but not least, to my fellow chocolate lovers, especially **Michelle**, who took me to the "dark side".

Dedication

My life has been shaped by those from whom I've learned...my family and friends, as well as those who also search for nutritional verities and educate about making responsible choices.

To my daughters who make me proud, and my siblings, parents and friends, for supporting my crazy ideas in tangible ways.

To the authors I admire for leading us to a better way - John Robbins, Neal Barnard, Howard Lyman, Sally Errey and others listed in the back of this book who have revolutionized our thinking and lifestyles. You've influenced and inspired my choices with your brilliant books, passing on knowledge and encouraging my confidence.

To Gerda and my other teachers for giving me the gift of yoga.

To my elders who taught and sacrificed with their example of dedication to family and community.

CONTENTS

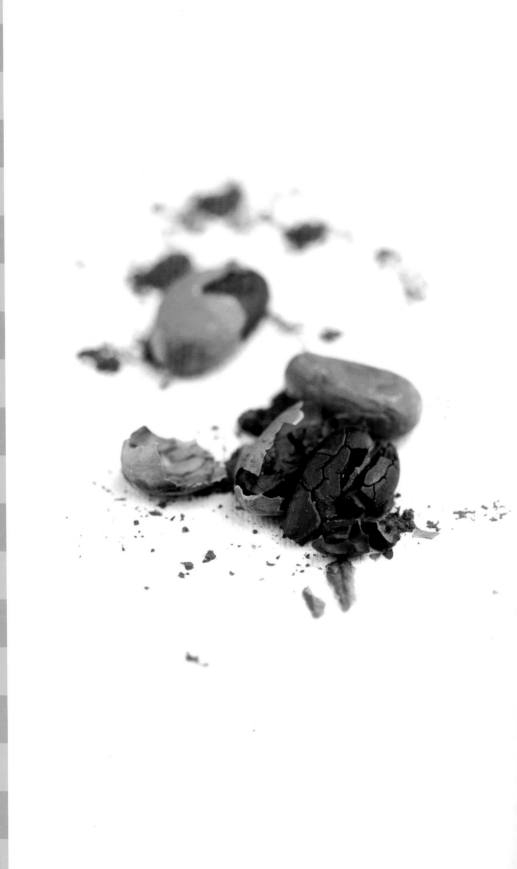

Foreword by John Robbins

It may surprise you to learn that chocolate is actually good for you. But it's true. There is a growing body of credible scientific evidence that chocolate contains a host of heart-healthy and mood-enhancing phytochemicals, with benefits to both body and mind.

For one thing, chocolate is a plentiful source of antioxidants. These are substances that reduce the ongoing cellular and arterial damage caused by oxidative reactions. Chocolate is particularly rich in a type of antioxidants called polyphenols. These are protective chemicals found in many plant foods, such as red wine and tea. According to researchers at the University of Texas Southwestern Medical Center in Dallas, the same antioxidant properties found in red wine that protect against heart disease and possibly cancer are also found in chocolate.

The oxidation of LDL cholesterol is a major risk factor in the promotion of coronary disease including heart attacks and strokes. When this waxy substance oxidizes, it tends to stick to artery walls, increasing the risk of a heart attack or stroke. The polyphenols in chocolate inhibit oxidation of LDL cholesterol.

One of the causes of atherosclerosis is blood platelets clumping together, a process called aggregation. The polyphenols in chocolate inhibit this clumping, reducing the risks of atherosclerosis.

People with heart problems are sometimes told to take a baby aspirin a day. The reason is that aspirin thins the blood and reduces the likelihood of clots forming (clots play a key role in many heart attacks and strokes). Research performed at the department of nutrition at the University of California, Davis, found that chocolate also thins the blood, and performs the same anti-clotting activity as aspirin. "Our work supports the concept that the chronic consumption of cocoa may be associated with improved cardiovascular health," said UC Davis researcher Carl Keen. "Cocoa and presumably other forms of chocolate can be part of a healthy diet."

How much chocolate would you have to eat to obtain these benefits? Not that much. According to a study published in the American Journal of Clinical Nutrition, adding half an ounce of dark chocolate to an average American diet increases total antioxidant capacity four percent, and lessens oxidation of LDL cholesterol.

What about the high levels of fat and sugar that we associate with chocolate products? This is certainly a concern. Nearly all of the calories in a typical chocolate bar, for example, are sugar and fat. But the primary fat in chocolate is stearic acid, and as far as fats go, it's not bad. It is a saturated vegetable fat, but unlike most saturated animal fats, stearic acid acts in the body much like the monounsaturated fat in olive oil. Monounsaturates have a neutral effect on cholesterol.

Watch out for milk chocolate, though, because it contains added butterfat which raises cholesterol, and it also contains cholesterol. (Cocoa butter, on the other hand is a vegetable fat, and so contains no cholesterol.) Milk chocolate has another disadvantage, too. It has less of the antioxidants and other beneficial chemicals than dark chocolate does.

Carob has a reputation as a more healthful substitute for chocolate. But in fact carob bars typically have more sugar than chocolate bars. One study at the University of Texas actually found carob bars to be five times more likely to cause tooth decay.

Most of us eat chocolate because we love the flavor, but chocolate is legendary as well for having effects on the mind. In fact, chocolate is so well known for its remarkable effects on human mood that some scientists consider it a psychoactive drug. Chocolate is the richest known source of a little-known substance called theobromine, a close chemical relative of caffeine. Theobromine, like caffeine, and also like the asthma drug theophylline, belong to the chemical group known as xanthine alkaloids. Chocolate products contain some caffeine, but not nearly enough to explain the attractions, fascinations, addictions, and effects of chocolate. Chocolate addiction may really be theobromine addiction.

Other substances with mood elevating effects are also found in chocolate. One is phenethylamine, which triggers the release of pleasurable endorphins and potentates the action of dopamine, a neurochemical associated with sexual arousal and pleasure. Phenethylamine is the chemical released in the brain when people become infatuated or fall in love. Another is anandamide (from the Sanskrit word "ananda," which means peaceful bliss). A fatty substance that is naturally produced in the brain, anandamide has been isolated from chocolate by pharmacologists at the Neurosciences Institute in San Diego. It binds to the same receptor sites in the brain as cannabinoids - the psychoactive constituents in marijuana, and produces feelings of euphoria.

If that weren't enough, chocolate also boosts brain levels of serotonin. Women typically have lower serotonin levels during PMS and menstruation, which may be one reason women typically experience stronger cravings for chocolate than men. People suffering from depression so characteristically have lower serotonin levels that an entire class of anti-depressive medications called serotonin uptake inhibitors (including Prozac, Paxil, and Zoloft) have been developed that raise brain levels of serotonin.

All this probably makes chocolate sound like a fabulous food, but please try to be aware of the fat and sugar in any chocolate products you might eat. Do I eat chocolate? Yes. Almost every day. Although after what I have learned about child slavery in the cocoa trade, I have a policy to eat only organic and/or fair trade chocolate. And I believe that anyone who eats chocolate should know about the current issue of child slavery in cocoa production. My article on this subject, titled **"Is There Slavery In Your Chocolate**," can be seen at **http://www.foodrevolution.org/slavery_chocolate.htm**.

May your life be full of healthy pleasures.

John Robbins, author
Healthy At 100, Diet For A New America,
The Food Revolution, and many other bestsellers

Foreword by Sally Errey

One of my missions in life is to help people feel good about food again. With most of our nutrition education coming from biased media advertisements it can be difficult to truly understand and make healthy choices. Finally, with Health By Chocolate, we have fantastic whole food recipes and ideas, supported by solid science, to make indulging in rich dark chocolate one of the most nutritious things to do each day! Now, eating quality chocolate is no longer a weakness but a strength!

Childhood, for most North Americans, is filled with sugary treats and junk food indulgences. The sight of a toddler's face covered in chocolate ice cream incites delight in all observers. Sadly, as we age the sweetness of these moments are lost to the reality of disease and illness. As adults we begin depriving ourselves of pleasurable foods in our quest for health and wellbeing. Fortunately, in this book, nutritionist Victoria Laine transforms this attitude of depravity into one of maturity. With recipes filled with nutrient rich ingredients that make delicious versions of the traditional, unhealthy variety, Victoria brings sweet indulgence back into a balanced diet.

The benefits of whole, natural unprocessed foods have been commented on for years and they are an integral part of my personal healthy eating plan and the fundamental basis for my own recipes and cookbooks. By combining everyone's favourite pleasure food, chocolate, with whole foods (which are loaded with beneficial nutrients, including phytochemicals, which help to prevent dis-ease and sustain us in a way processed foods never will) Victoria has created recipes that bring nourishment to both body and soul.

Life is hard. You endeavour to live each day without regrets. And on your deathbed you may wish you had laughed more, worried less, eaten better; but now, thanks to Health by Chocolate, it is doubtful that you will think, "I wish I had eaten less chocolate!"

Sally Errey, R.H.N, R.N.C.P.

Nutrition Consultant, speaker, and best selling author of
Staying Alive! Cookbook for Cancer Free Living
Rooibos Revolution - Recipes for Nature's Healing Tea

HEALTH & HAPPINESS
BY CHOCOLATE

In **HEALTH by CHOCOLATE: Radical New Recipes & Nutrition Know-How** you'll embark on a journey of discovery that will surprise and delight you! Learn of the many sides of chocolate – its chemistry and nutrition, its sensuality and humour, and even your purchasing power of the 'food of the gods'. You will be treated to delicious, easy to prepare chocolate recipes that you and your friends can enjoy with guilt-free pleasure and healthy satisfaction. From quick and simple smoothies, dairy-free ice cream and cheesecake to energy bars, brownies and mousse, the choices are abundant. Family and friends will be impressed, looking forward with excited anticipation when you whip up the next creation for a daily snack, meal-on-the-run or special treat.

The mood enhancing and hormonal benefits of chocolate are what led me to a passionate investigation of this seductive topic. My interest began when a traumatic experience toppled my world and threatened to spiral me into a deep depression. My chocolate consumption escalated from a few ounces several times a week to an obvious addiction. Now I've wisely come to depend on at least one daily dose of healthy quality chocolate.

In my nutritional practice I encounter many clients who struggle with chocolate desires, addiction and guilt. Once I begin sharing healthy chocolate recipes to satisfy their chocolate cravings, I see a higher rate of compliance in their overall dietary changes. I recommend they continue their chocolate habit, yet enjoy only the healthiest choices. They are delighted, often ecstatic to learn they don't have to eliminate chocolate from their diets. It is a win-win situation. They are still able to lose weight, balance blood sugars, lower cholesterol and triglycerides, and continue to enjoy delicious and easy to prepare treats.

The concern nutritionists have with chocolate is the amount of added sugar and total fat that is part of the chocolate experience. The daily caloric intake of sugar and fat is important, but **the types of sugars and fats consumed are also crucial to health.** Learning to partner healthy chocolate with a meal plan that includes sufficient fibre-filled and enzyme-rich veggies, fruits, whole grains, and legumes (beans) means discovering that chocolate is no longer forbidden or guilt inducing.

Compiling this book, I delved into the latest research on the health benefits of cocoa. I also discovered the history of, and production of chocolate, as well as the politics and ethics of one of the most appealing flavours in the world. There is more to know about this little bean than I ever imagined. I've focused mainly on nutrition and health factors of eating chocolate, and **included a Healthy Chocolate Kitchen Guide and Ingredient Glossary. 'From Cacao Bean to Chocolate Bar'** will further guide you in your chocolate choices. You can refer to the excellent resource list at the back of this book for more information on whole food nutrition and other aspects of chocolate.

My motivation in writing this book is to educate readers on the nutritional benefits of chocolate and whole foods, and provide truly healthful chocolate recipes that are quick and easy to make. If you're ready to incorporate healthy choices into your repertoire, prepare to dive into some delicious, delightful 'radical new chocolate recipes'! Try some chocolate for breakfast - yes BREAKFAST - and you'll start your day right!!

Many friends, family members, clients and students have awaited the completion of this book with less-than-patient anticipation. I can think of no other indulgent fare that elicits such passionate responses as chocolate.

You know the adage – "When life hands you lemons, make lemonade"? Well, I've translated that into – "When life hands you bitter lumps and bumps, make sweet, smooth chocolate recipes!" And here they are, packed with pure pleasure and filled with natural goodness, so we can enjoy them free of guilt.

HEALTH by CHOCOLATE: Radical New Recipes & Nutrition Know-How will delight your taste buds, support your immune system, turn up your brain power and make your heart healthy and happy! How can you resist something this seductive?

As Hippocrates said:

'Let our food be our medicine, and our medicine be our food'…so let's raise our cocoa mugs to the "food of the gods"…and let the healing begin!!

FOR THE LOVE OF CHOCOLATE
The Moods and Minds of
CHOCOLATE LOVERS and CHOCOHOLICS

Don't stop to think…just fill in the blank with whatever comes to mind.

Chocolate is _____

These are some comments clients and friends have declared about chocolate.

~ Chocolate is "to die for". ~ Chocolate heals a broken heart.
~ Chocolate is sinful. ~ Chocolate is my life. ~ Chocolate is my downfall.
~ Chocolate is heavenly/divine. ~ Chocolate gives me acne.
~ Chocolate equals relief! ~ Chocolate is better than sex.
~ Chocolate is my best friend. ~ I shamefully admit
to my chocolate addiction. ~ Chocolate is my medicine.
~ Chocolate is orgasmic. ~ Chocolate is my saving grace.
~ Chocolate makes me fat. ~ Chocolate is "inner warmth".

Chocolate evokes a host of thoughts and responses. The attitudes and beliefs about chocolate can be contradictory, leaving us in a state of confusion or guilt. Why does feeling bad become associated with something that gives us such pleasure? With a clear understanding of how to use chocolate healthfully, we can enjoy the delights of chocolate, letting go of negativity.

Used wisely, partnered with whole food ingredients, chocolate is a delicious and healthy choice.

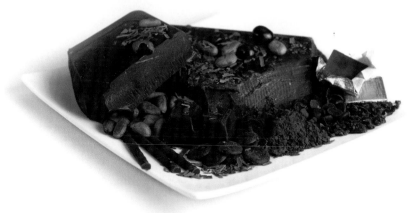

CONFESSIONS OF AN ADDICTED NUTRITION COUNSELLOR

(or…How I got hooked on the most delicious "drug of choice"!)

I had struggled with my health from an early age. As a child and teen I suffered from frequent colds and infections. In my early adult years I learned that allergies and food sensitivities were the reason for these symptoms and I began to make changes to my diet. One of the foods suggested as being a potential trigger was chocolate so, along with other foods, I completely stopped eating it. For several years I didn't touch even a morsel. (I was yet to learn that food sensitivity could potentially resolve after a short abstinence of the trigger(s) and some digestive healing.) In those days all chocolate was blacklisted by health food nuts, (like myself) as "junk food", because the health benefits of chocolate were largely unknown.

Writing a book on chocolate and promoting its use makes the self-imposed deprivation I sustained for so long, quite ironic! As the years went by, my overall health improved. With the emerging news of the nutritional benefits of chocolate, I decided it couldn't be that bad to allow myself small amounts of a high quality chocolate occasionally.

My "now and then" habit gradually became an almost daily occurrence as I drew closer to menopause. One day in yoga class, one of my students shared what another yoga instructor had said. "I eat a small piece of dark quality chocolate every day, to remind myself that life is sweet." I LOVED that idea. How symbolic and, well… sweet! It is important to remember, I thought, especially in the tough times, how sweet and precious life is. I decided then I would give up my guilt over the daily chocolate consumption and continue "using" it.

After years of personal investigation and reading about nutrition and wellness, I received formal education and finally turned my passion for healthy food preparation and its benefits into a career as a holistic nutrition counsellor and teacher.

Working with clients and over the years, watching women (and some men) inhale chocolate as though their lives depended on it, I've been curious about its mood-altering and hormonal affects. The guilt so many women carry about their relationship to this "food of the gods", as it's historically referred to, is also a curiosity. How can we receive such pleasure and at the same time feel such guilt from consuming it? Is chocolate really a food, or should it more accurately be considered a drug? We know it has mood-enhancing effects because of the chemicals that release endorphins, and those that stimulate production of the "feel-good" brain chemical, serotonin.

Confessions of many female clients' boundless passion for chocolate has highlighted for me how intense women's love affair with chocolate really is. Certainly there are males who are just as crazy about chocolate, but it seems that females are more likely to become "addicted".

I've joined the ranks of those who use chocolate as their "drug of choice". On hearing news of this book project, one friend started calling me a "cocoa pushing drug lord". I smiled and offered her another truffle!

An Affair with Chocolate

Chocolate helped me to deal with the experience that has been the most painful and difficult time in my life, in a way I would not have thought possible. I noticed that while I often felt depressed in the morning, soon after I'd eaten some chocolate in the afternoon, my mood and energy picked up and the rest of the day became manageable. I decided to experiment with a dose (or two) of chocolate in the mornings. When I did, I found it made a significant difference; it boosted my spirits enough to get me through the morning hours more easily. I managed to deal with this devastating experience without the use of antidepressants (or any other potentially addictive chemical). Along with the love and support from cherished friends and family, prayer and chocolate got me through those difficult days. Chocolate therapy aided my healing. I clearly understand now why chocolate is considered "divine".

THE UPSIDE, DOWNSIDE, LIGHTSIDE AND DARKSIDE OF THE "FOOD OF THE GODS"

The history, nutritional benefits, chemistry, consumption and consumerism of chocolate are truly fascinating. Here is a bit of what I've learned and love to share with others.

Cacao has been used for centuries as a tonic to lift moods and improve endurance. It's been long known that cacao (Latin: theobroma cacao) has chemicals that create mood-enhancing hormonal effects. The claims for cocoa's benefits range from its "feel good" effects to its potential to improve heart health, and to help prevent cancer. Historically, people appreciated its health building benefits:

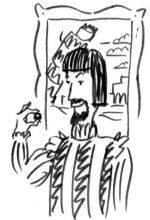

▶ Cocoa was first used as a beverage, mixed with water. The Aztec emperor, Montezuma (c.1480-1520) believed cocoa was "the divine drink, which builds up resistance and fights fatigue. A cup of this precious drink permits a man to walk for a whole day without food."

▶ An Italian physician, Stephani Blancardi (1650-1702) believed "chocolate is not only pleasant of taste, but it is also a veritable balm of the mouth, for the maintaining of all glands and humours in a good state of health."

Is it all good news? Is chocolate a cure-all, a miracle drug? Are all chocolate product created equally? Let's look at some of the present day understanding.

THE UPSIDE...HAPPY HAPPY HORMONES!

A HEALTHY HIGH with CHOCOLATE

Chocolate is often used when we're under stress. Perhaps it is being used now more than ever, to help us cope with the "rat race" lifestyle of so many today. It can be a valuable aide for lifting spirits and improving endurance during stressful times.

The mood-enhancing benefits and chocolate's pleasurable effects are due to bioactive substances such as tryptophan, phenethylamine and theobromine in the cocoa that trigger serotonin (a neurotransmitter involved in regulating moods). Some research has suggested that opiate-like substances in cocoa can trigger a dopamine release (a neurotransmitter and precursor to adrenaline) in the brain.

Brain chemistry is complex and it may not be completely understood why some people find chocolate more pleasurable, even more "addictive" than others. Many herbalists and nutritionists consider cocoa a hormone-enhancing food for women. There are theories as to why so many women have an intimate relationship with chocolate, the cravings associated with PMS and menopause, perhaps future research will be able to fully explain this link.

Some scientists and clinicians hypothesize that food cravings are the body's way of correcting a nutritional deficiency. Others argue that non-chocolate foods containing the same substances would also satisfy the craving. For example, chocolate is considered to be high in magnesium, so if a magnesium deficiency is present, other foods high in magnesium would satisfy the craving, but this is not the case. There is something uniquely attractive that drives people to chocolate. Studies done in 2000 found neuroactive alkaloids that are naturally present in alcohol, are also found in small quantities in cocoa, leading researchers to consider how these compounds may be related to addiction. No conclusive evidence is available to completely explain cravings.

Although addictive behaviour is usually associated with drugs and alcohol – and in no way should the seriousness of these destructive addictions be minimized – chocolate has, in the minds of many, become linked to "addiction". Many people, especially women, pride themselves on their "chocoholism", openly admitting their crazed passion. Then there are the "closet chocoholics" who only reveal their "deep dark secret" when it's coaxed from them.

Next time you want to "get high"…consider this:

> *"I can recommend switching to chocolate for all you addictive types… Think of the advantages …chocolate doesn't make you stupid and clumsy. It doesn't render you incapable of operating heavy machinery…You don't have to smuggle chocolate across the border…Possession, even possession with intent to sell, is perfectly legal…and second-hand chocolate doesn't offend the people around you."*
>
> Linda Henley (b.1951 American columnist)
> *Chocolate: The Exquisite Indulgence* © 1995 by Running Press

Of course, there are other mood-enhancing practices like exercise, music, art, laughter, chanting, meditation and prayer that alter brain chemistry and can act as mood elevators. While these practices are highly recommended and an important part of my own lifestyle, in my opinion, chocolate is in a realm of its own. Perhaps this is only because its indulgence takes such little effort!

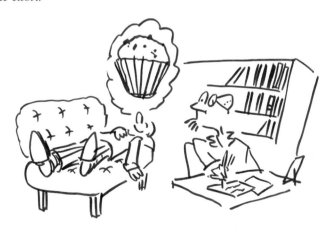

Chocolate and Yoga: A Match Made in Heaven

Joy upon joy, bliss upon bliss! To practice yoga under the influence of chocolate is something "out of this world". Yoga, in and of itself, can be uplifting. With a focus on bringing oxygen to the brain, increasing circulation and creating endorphins, yoga is a great way to lift our moods. But add a dose of chocolate to the experience and we're heading for a retreat from stress that can't help but change our outlook on life…at least for a while. As temporary as the "fix" may be, we can always look forward to the next chocolate-yoga experience, and know there is a sweet, delicious way to lift out of gloominess. The same goes for other uplifting practices like prayer, laughter and music; add chocolate to these experiences…and life becomes heavenly.

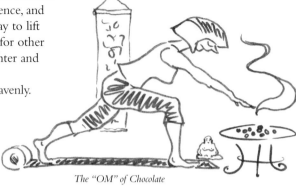

The "OM" of Chocolate

Chocolate Laughter Therapy

Have you ever heard of Laughter Yoga? Laughter Clubs have cropped up all over the world. "Laugh yourself healthy" is the motto of the clubs. It is a series of yogic breathing and movement exercises designed to stimulate laughter without the use of humor or jokes. The worldwide laughter movement started in India in 1995 when Dr. Madan Kataria, a Mumbai physician, discovered the physical and psychological benefits enjoyed by his patients who had taken to heart his prescription for regular laughter. Laughter was the healing strategy used by Norman Cousins, author of **Anatomy of an Illness**, who after being diagnosed with a life threatening illness was cured with high doses of vitamin C and a regimen of daily doses of belly laughter. Try a potent combination of a dose of laughter and chocolate to chase away the blues!

A Chocolate Meditation

One of the opportunities I offer my students at the end of a yoga class, is a few minutes of breathing deeply along with taking "a gratitude moment"…to think of someone or something they are grateful for today.

It may be that you don't practice yoga, but have a special time of the day (maybe first thing in the morning or last thing at night) where you cherish a special conversation or event that took place recently. Perhaps you take time each day to pray, for yourself or others, asking for guidance or giving thanks.

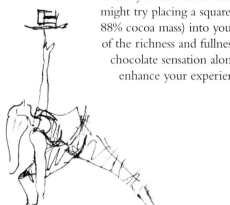

When you take those moments for retreat, renewal or celebration, you might try placing a square of dark nutritious chocolate (my favourite is a 88% cocoa mass) into your mouth, close your eyes and remind yourself of the richness and fullness life offers. Enjoy the deep pleasure of the chocolate sensation along with 'being in the moment'. Perhaps it will enhance your experience of connecting to the Divine!

~ Namaste

THE NUTRITION OF CHOCOLATE

I'm fairly certain that if we took a poll we'd find that most people don't consume chocolate on the basis of its scientifically proven health-enhancing effects or nutritional benefits…but for its delicious, sensuous taste and "feel good" expression. So while cocoa may be getting a lot of press recently due to the newly discovered phytochemicals, let's not lose sight of the fact that it's always had a great reputation. Partaking of chocolate will continue to be motivated by that deep inner knowing that, "It'll make me feel better."

However, it is important to understand is that there is "chocolate"…and then there is CHOCOLATE! One choice can negatively impact our health, while another can positively enhance our health. So if we're going to use it regularly…let's do it right!

MICRO and MACRO NUTRIENTS IN CHOCOLATE (Cacao beans, cacao nibs, cocoa powder and products made from them)

▶ Cacao contains essential minerals - magnesium, iron, calcium, phosphorus, zinc, copper, potassium, and manganese - as well as some vitamins.

▶ Cacao also contains protein (5-15%), complex carbohydrate (20-50%) and soluble dietary fibre (5-20%), depending on the degree of processing. Cacao beans and nibs contain about 50% fat. Cocoa powder has much of the cacao butter (fat) removed when processed and usually only contains between 10-25% fat. Manufacturers add back cacao butter to quality cooking chocolate and chocolate bars that results in a creamier texture.

▶ Cacao butter has a number of qualities, some of them controversial. It is about two-thirds saturated fat in the form of stearic, oleic and palmitic acids. Although saturated fat has a reputation for being unhealthy and leading to heart disease, it is becoming apparent that the saturated fats in plant foods are different than from those in animal foods. The stearic acid in cocoa butter does not raise levels of LDL cholesterol in the bloodstream, and in fact some studies indicate it may actually lower them. Milk fats and other processed fats added to chocolate products can, however, adversely affect lipid and cholesterol levels.

▶ Cacao butter is the only vegetable fat that melts at a point just below body temperature; this gives it that beautiful "melt in your mouth" creamy sensation, and explains my present daily addiction to truffles.

ANTIOXIDANTS

Much research has been done into the heart health benefits as well as potential anti-cancer action of naturally occurring compounds. Recent scientific study has shown a number of valuable cocoa compounds not previously recognized. Antioxidants counter the "free radical action" in our cells that contribute to aging and disease. Antioxidants measurements are rated by ORAC (Oxygen Radical Absorbance Capacity) values and more recently by TAC (Total Anti-oxidant Capacity).

FLAVANOLS…for the CHOCOLATE LOVER'S HEALTHY HEART ♥

The Kuna Indians of Panama are heavy consumers of flavanol rich, raw cocoa, and drink 3-5 cups daily as well as consuming raw cacao in other dishes. The incidence of death from heart attacks, strokes, diabetes and cancer is considerably lower in comparison of the Kuna Indians who moved to the mainland and discontinued their use of the daily cocoa beverages.

Many chocolate studies now making headlines are funded by chocolate interest groups and large cocoa companies. Independent studies of the health advantages of cocoa are not as abundant. However, these too confirm many of the antioxidant benefits of the flavanols present in pure cocoa. In the book, **Foods That Fight Cancer,** authors Richard Béliveau,

Ph.D. and Denis Gingras, Ph.D. report encouraging results of anti-cancer properties in early studies, due to the abundance of polyphenols (300 mg in 50 g) in dark chocolate.

Cocoa's flavanols (procyanidins) are believed to boost blood flow, due to increased nitric oxide bioavailability to the heart, brain, and other parts of the body. They can also suppress inflammatory responses that are associated with heart health, and suppress the tendency for blood clot formation.

The flavanols may have the potential, in sufficient quantities, to reduce high blood pressure, heart disease, some cancers and even learning and memory challenges. (Just remember to take your chocolate!) However some of the flavanols are lost in the processing of the raw cocoa meat or "nib" into cocoa powder and cocoa products. The alkali used in "Dutch processed" cocoa powder production renders the antioxidant flavanols less available.

Flavanols have received a great deal of attention recently, as the antioxidants in pure cocoa are known to be higher than those in green tea, red wine and blueberries. Dark chocolate is much higher in flavanols than many veggies and fruits, at 826 TAC units per gram. Of course, it is advisable to consume more calories from fruits and vegetables than from chocolate!

THE DOWNSIDE...TURNED RIGHT-SIDE UP!

There is a vast difference between low quality, inferior chocolate and high quality, superior, dark chocolate. The former must be regarded "junk" food, while the latter, chosen well, can undoubtedly be considered "nutritious".

Abundantly available in vending machines and convenience stores, low quality chocolate confectionery is probably one of the leading causes, along with soda pop, of obesity and diabetes. If the North American pandemics of diabetes and obesity, cardiovascular dis-ease and cancers are ever going to be addressed from a preventative approach, people have to embrace truly healthy nutritional practices that are supported with honest, accurate nutritional information for consumers. Governments are responsible for educating the public and ensuring accurate nutritional labelling to empower consumers. Non-profit, non-governmental agencies like Physicians Committee For Responsible Medicine (PCRM), (see Resources) are proactively affecting positive change in the way present day health and diet are viewed.

Where we run into trouble is when we consume chocolate products with LOW QUALITY PROCESSED INGREDIENTS (eg. refined sugars and corn syrups, milk fats, milk solids, hydrogenated fats, food colouring, flavours, preservatives and other "non-food" ingredients like waxy parathons), many of which have been linked to various health concerns.

Low quality chocolate bars and foodstuffs contain lower amounts of the nutrient-rich cocoa and higher amounts of empty calories. The majority of the chocolate eaten today is made inexpensively with damaging features out-weighing any nutritional benefits. High quality chocolate products use high percentages of pure cocoa ingredients, partnered with other nutrient-rich ingredients.

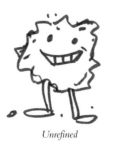

Unrefined   *Refined*

Refined sugars are considered by nutritionists to be "anti-nutrients" because they leave a defici on our nutritional score sheet. Non-nutritive "sugar-free" sweeteners (like aspartame) are the topic of much debate. There have been reports of negative side effects from popular sugar substitutes that include a multitude of concerns, including severe nervous system damage. There is also <u>no</u> evidence that they assist in weight loss or blood sugar balancing as they are alleged to do. For more in-depth information on sugar, see **Defeating Diabetes** and **Excitotoxins: The Taste That Kills** (see Resources).

Transfats and other damaged fats still used in processed foods and low quality confectionery chocolate are damaging to our cells by creating free radicals. They should be avoided and replaced with fresh fats in whole foods and raw oils, like those found in the recipes in this book.

COCOA PARTNERS

Why not DAIRY?

Dairy, legumes (beans), and nuts/seeds are three main food group sources of amino acids (protein) and essential fatty acids (fat). Allergies can develop to any of these sources and are most likely from milk, soy, and nuts. Dairy allergy and lactose intolerance is prevalent in the population. This is one reason dairy ingredients are not included in these recipes.

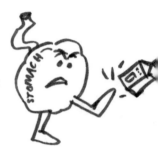

Visit the **P.C.R.M. Healthy School Lunches** website (see Resources) to learn more about the issue of dairy intolerance, including the following statistics

"According to the American Academy of Family Physicians' 2002 report on lactose intolerance, 60 percent to 80 percent of blacks, 50 percent to 80 percent of Hispanics, 80 percent to 100 percent of American Indians, 95 percent to 100 percent of Asians, and 6 percent to 22 percent of American whites are lactose intolerant. Lactose intolerance, which is sometimes apparent as early as age three, causes flatulence, cramping, diarrhea, and bloating after eating dairy products."

Processed milk products are commonly used in confectionery chocolate and poor quality commercially produced foods.

There are other reasons dairy foods are being eliminated from many peoples' diet. Dairy products are mucus forming and contribute to digestive challenges. Even organic versions of dairy products contain natural growth hormones (meant for speedy growth of calves) that have been linked to human weight challenges. Read **MILK A-Z** (see Resources) for a startling compilation of scientific reasons to minimize or eliminate dairy foods from your diet. As well, livestock are reported by the United Nations Food and Agriculture Organization to be "one o the most significant contributors to today's most serious environmental problems …a major source of land and water degradation".

So SOY?

Soy has significant heart health and anti-cancer benefits. Tofu is known as a good source of isoflavones, believed to relieve hot flashes in menopausal women. While some tofu in the diet is healthful, as people are switching from dairy to soy and the marketplace is supplying an abundance of processed soy products, many have no resemblance to the mighty whole soy bean. Eating an excess of soy, especially large amounts of highly processed soy, may pose health concerns. Too much soy may suppress thyroid function, and especially should not be used in excess; no more than one to two servings per day if you have a thyroid condition. Always use a variety of legumes (beans) in your diet. Use tofu along with fermented soy (e.g. tempeh, miso, natto) as these provide digestive benefits. For more helpful information on soy, go to **www.foodrevolution.org/what_about_soy.htm**

Got NUTS? Many nuts and seeds provide similar protein, carbohydrate and fat profiles to dairy foods, but they also provide dietary fibres that dairy foods do not. Like all animal products, dairy foods are completely devoid of fibre. Nuts and seeds contain essential fatty acids that dairy foods do not. When nuts and seeds are consumed raw, lightly toasted, or sprouted, they provide beneficial enzymes. Milk (both dairy and soy), when pasteurized, contains no enzymes. Nut-meats are also high in antioxidant nutrients. Nuts and seeds can make surprisingly 'creamy' replacements for milk and dairy products. Look for delicious, nut-milk and nut-milk smoothies in this book. Again, variety is important both for nutrient availability and food rotation so as to prevent allergic conditions. Nuts and seeds provide essential nutrients like fatty acids, enzymes, protein, complex carbohydrate, fibre, antioxidant vitamins and minerals - magnesium, iron, potassium, selenium, copper and zinc. Nuts and seeds are low on the glycemic index.

Studies on the heart-protective benefits of nuts have shown conclusive results that nuts should be an important, regular part of a wholefoods diet. Eating nut-meats is also linked to lower risk of diabetes, some cancers, and macular degeneration, as well as longevity according to authors Liz Pearson, R.D. and Mairlyn Smith, H.Ec. in **Ultimate Foods for Ultimate Health...and don't forget the chocolate!**

WHAT ABOUT NATURALLY OCCURRING COMPOUNDS?

Is Chocolate high in Caffeine? Many people think chocolate is a high source of caffeine. In fact, caffeine, a stimulant to those who are sensitive, is present in relatively low amounts in cocoa. (While an 8 ounce (220mL) cup of coffee contains 100-150mL of caffeine, a same size cup of cocoa contains only 15 mL of caffeine and one ounce of solid bittersweet chocolate has a mere 5-10 mL of caffeine.) Theobromine, a chemical in cocoa that is of the same family as caffeine, also increases alertness without making the heart and nerves jittery like caffeine can.

Does chocolate prevent dental caries? Research at Tulane University in New Orleans found theobromine (a white powder extracted from cacao) to be even more effective than flouride in fighting cavities, causing it to be considered as an additive to toothpaste.

How does chocolate affect bone density? Cacao contains oxalates, naturally occurring compounds, which in large quantities are considered to inhibit calcium absorption. Oxalates are also found in varying amounts in rhubarb, spinach, sweet potatoes, kale, collards, chard, okra, berries and tea. The amount of oxalate in cacao is small. The new research at Tulane University also indicates a bone bolstering affect from the theobromine present in chocolate. Chocolate is high in magnesium and phosphorus, two other bone building minerals. Pairing your chocolate (and other foods containing oxalates) with sesame seeds, almonds, dark leafy greens, tofu and other calcium rich foods is a helpful way to ensure more minerals are present in your diet.

Cocoa is naturally high in copper, and copper excess may lead to opposing mineral deficiencies and inhibit the action of some flavanoids, particularly hesperidin. Ensure your diet is high in minerals by including vegetables that have been grown in mineral rich soil, and sea vegetables such a kelp and dulse.

Does Chocolate Cause Acne? Chocolate has previously been considered a factor of acne. The antioxidants in pure cocoa are actually known to help develop a healthy complexion. Studies have shown that even frequent consumption of cocoa has no effect on the outbreak of acne. It is more likely the inferior sugars and milk ingredients that lead to deficiencies or excesses that produce acne.

THE LIGHTSIDE...BECOMING "EN-LIGHT-ENED"!

CHOOSING HEALTHFUL CHOCOLATE

The best way to get on the good side of chocolate is to purchase products (like bars and ready-made goodies) that use only premium grade chocolate and only whole food ingredients.

Or, make your own delicious snacks, meals, treats and desserts, like those found in the recipes in Part 2 of this book. You can easily learn to partner quality pure cocoa (including melting-chocolate) with whole food ingredients for optimum nutrition and flavours. The healthiest chocolate products and recipes are those that use whole cacao, cacao nibs and cocoa powder combined with the healthiest added ingredients.

For more guidance on the educated purchasing and healthy consumption of cocoa and chocolate see FROM CACAO BEAN TO CHOCOLATE BAR, and THE HEALTHY CHOCOLATE KITCHEN GUIDE (Part 2).

QUALITY and QUANTITY

Whole food chocolate products are loaded with health building nutrients, so appropriate portions are more likely to satiate with fewer calories, potentially giving us control over how much we consume.

WHAT ARE WHOLE FOODS?

Whole foods and whole food ingredients:

▶ are as close to their natural state as possible;

▶ have not been highly processed or refined (like white flour and white sugar have), or altered in ways that significantly decrease their nutritional value;

▶ have not had anything taken away, or added to them (eg. bran and germ removed from grains, or preservatives added) to decrease their quality;

▶ are nutritionally dense and health enhancing

▶ include whole grains, legumes, vegetables, fruits, nuts and seeds.

There is clear evidence that a simple, whole food, plant based, balanced diet can prevent and sometimes even reverse heart disease and diabetes. It's exciting to see the healing power of food, along with other healthy habits, reverse type 2 diabetes, high cholesterol and triglycerides, high blood pressure, and obesity using this whole foods diet, often within only a matter of months.

A WORD ABOUT FIBRE...

Animal foods (including eggs and dairy) are devoid of fibre, and plant foods contain varying amounts of fibre. In order to get sufficient daily fibre (a minimum of 35-50 grams), one needs to eat, predominately, a variety of plant foods - whole grains, legumes (beans), veggies, fruit, nuts and seeds.

A WORD ABOUT ENZYMES...

Food enzymes are essential to health. Enzymes are considered "the spark of life", and are catalysts for vitamins and minerals. Enzymes are available in raw fruits, vegetables, nuts and seeds, and sprouted legumes and grains. Enzymes are destroyed when heated past 118°F. Include a high percentage of raw foods in your diet for optimum nutrition.

QUALITY SWEETENERS

Whole cacao beans and pure cocoa powder are bitter, so the sweetness of chocolate depends on what amount and form of sweetener is added to the cocoa (see Table 1) and THE HEALTHY CHOCOLATE KITCHEN GUIDE (Part 2).

For sufficient energy, most active people require between 55 and 65% of their daily calories from carbohydrate. All carbohydrates (simple or complex), whether from refined sugars or whole food sources, are broken down by digestion into simple sugars that become blood glucose and either act as energy or are stored as fat. However, not all sugars are created equally. So why are we wise to choose "natural sugars" over refined and processed ones? One difference is the micro-nutrient values. Typically, the more processed a food is, the more micro-nutrients and phytochemicals are destroyed, so fewer vitamins and minerals are available, whereas nutrient dense foods naturally retain vitamins and minerals, and possibly fibre and food enzymes.

In these recipes, fruits, nut-meats and seeds provide natural sweetness (in the form of simple and complex carbohydrates), and most provide a good source of dietary fibre. If they are in their raw state, they also have enzymatic benefits needed for many cellular and digestive functions. While some natural sweeteners (eg. honey, maple syrup, agave nectar, brown rice syrup) are not high in fibre, they provide other health building nutrients. If you are diabetic or struggle with blood sugar swings, choose recipes that contain fruits, nuts or seeds over those with fibreless sugars, as both the fibre and the fat help to slow the metabolism of the carbohydrates into the bloodstream. Nuts and seeds are rich in complex carbohydrates that help to keep blood sugar balanced and energy steady.

TABLE 1: NUTRITIONAL PROFILE FOR COMPARISON (100 grams)

	Maple Syrup	Honey	Blackstrap Molasses	Dates	Refined Sugar
Calories	261	304	235	282	387
Fat	0.2 g			0.39 g	
Sodium	9 mg	4 mg	55 mg	2 mg	2 mg
Potassium	204 mg	52 mg	2492 mg	656 mg	99.98 g
Carbohydrates	67.09 g	82.4 g	60.8 g	75.03 g	
Dietary Fibre		0.2 g		8 g	
Protein		0.3 g		2.45 g	
Vitamin A				10 IU	
Vitamin C		0.5 mg		0.4 mg	
Calcium	67 mg	6 mg	860 mg	39 mg	1 mg
Iron	1.2 mg	0.42 mg	17.5 mg	1.02 mg	
Thiamine			0.03 mg	0.05 mg	
Riboflavin		0.04 mg	0.05 mg	0.07 mg	0.02mg
Niacin	0.03 mg	0.12 mg	1.08 mg	1.27 mg	
Vitamin B6		0.02 mg	0.7 mg	0.17 mg	
Folate		2 µg	1 µg	19 µg	
Pantothenic Acid	0.04 mg	0.07 mg	0.88 mg	0.59 mg	
Phosphorus	2 mg	4 mg	40 mg	62 mg	
Magnesium	14 mg	2 mg	215 mg	43 mg	
Zinc	4.16 mg	0.22 mg	1 mg	0.29 mg	
Copper	0.07 mg	0.04 mg	2.04 mg	0.21 mg	
Manganese	3.30 mg	0.08 mg	2.61 mg	0.26 mg	
Selenium	0.6 µg	0.8 µg	17.8 µg	3 µg	0.6 µg
Water	32.11 mg	17.1 mg	28.70 mg	20.53 mg	0.03 mg

U.S.D.A. SR-16

QUALITY FATS

When it comes to discerning "appropriate amounts" of fats, keep in mind that most people need between 20 and 30% of their daily calories from fat. Fat gives flavour to food, slows digestion and the release of sugar into the bloodstream, as well as helping us feel satiated. Fatty acids, provided in whole food fats, are crucial for our hormonal system, immune system, brain function and other cellular needs. A deficiency of healthy fats can result in dry skin, brittle nails and hair, hormonal imbalance and other health concerns, while an excess can show up as weight gain, high blood pressure, liver strain and hormonal imbalance.

Processed oils sold in bottles, and packaged products that sit on shelves for lengthy periods, have reduced amounts of nutrients. They may also contain deodorizers to mask the rancidity or chemical preservatives necessary to keep them shelf stable. Raw fats on the other hand, found in whole foods (like nuts, seeds and avocados) as well as expeller-pressed oils sold in refrigerated bottles, have superior nutrition, providing an abundance of antioxidant vitamins and minerals.

Are nuts high in calories? Yes, there is a range of fat and calories in nuts and seeds, some very high in calories and some that are comparable to other common food choices. Fat provides more calories per gram (9) than carbohydrate and protein (4). Once thought to be too "high calorie", nutmeats were recommended to be avoided completely. Used in appropriate amounts however, along with a balance of other whole foods, they can be a healthy choice. Some of the lowest fat sources are almonds, cashews, peanuts, pistachios, and sunflower, pumpkin, sesame, hemp and flax seeds. Highest fat sources are macadamias, pecans and Brazil nuts, which should be kept to a minimum or avoided if you are on a weight reduction diet. When consumed, pair with high fibre meals.

DOES CHOCOLATE CAUSE WEIGHT GAIN?

A regular chocolate habit can cause weight gain, but it doesn't have to! This book was designed with nutrient density as the key, and flavour satisfaction as the goal. Of course, eating calories in excess of your activity level can lead to weight gain. However, when you are eating a diet of three balanced meals, of mostly or completely whole plant foods (whole grains, legumes, veggies, and fruits), you can give yourself permission to enjoy an appropriate amount of these calorie and nutrient dense recipes with sheer pleasure, savouring each delicious morsel.

High Calorie Insanity! Some of the recipes in this book may be considered "high" in calories, or fat…but wait…is that a bad thing? Let's take a rational look at this issue. We all require a certain number of calories to maintain our health and energy - for adults usually between 1,200 and 3,000 depending on activity levels. Where we get those calories is what matters. For example, if we eat commercial, low quality foods (including chocolate products), we get low amounts of vitamins, minerals and micronutrients, but if we consume high quality whole food ingredients, we obtain high amounts of vitamins, minerals, enzymes and fibres. Same number of calories…but with superior nutritional advantage. When ingredients are fibre-filled, we feel fuller faster, so we may actually consume many fewer calories than from a similar recipe of traditionally processed ingredients. We get the delicious tastes and flavours with high nutrient value, so our taste buds are happy and so is our body. I recently heard a television chef exclaim that he got his nutrition from his healthy meals, not from his desserts. You will learn, in this book, just how easy it is to get high nutrition value from your desserts too. No more empty calories!

How much is too much? Identifying how much is appropriate consumption can be challenging. The interpretation of moderation varies from person to person, so "eat in moderation" amounts to vague advice. Interestingly, just as I was completing this manuscript, I was presented with a delightful book by Chloe Doutre-Roussel called **Chocolate Connoisseur**, in which the author, an amazing 5'3" woman and famous chocolate buyer for a major European store, states that she eats at least one pound of quality chocolate daily (mostly in the form of premium grade dark chocolate bars), and maintains her weight at 100-105 lbs! She is active, swims an hour a day and enjoys a healthy lifestyle. Not everyone's rate of metabolism is the same, but certainly regular exercise is an important contributor to building and maintaining healthy metabolism.

Half of a 3 oz/85 g dark (72%) chocolate bar contains 220 calories (providing 11% of a 2,000 calorie diet), which is about 25% of our daily fat requirement. If we double that and eat the entire bar in a day, we really should make up the rest of our calories with beans and veggies instead of steak and eggs, to be sure! Cocoa powder contains the phytochemical and anti-oxidant benefits with less fat calories than chocolate ingredients containing full cocoa butter.

I believe it's important that we mindfully savour instead of mindlessly devour our food, including our chocolate. I think it wise to serve our family and guests small portions of rich treats, no matter how nutrient dense, enabling them to gauge their "fullness factor" without the pressure of overeating just to be polite (of course, second helpings can be available to those who desire).

Keep in mind also that, chemically speaking, anything used in excess can potentially reverse the effect of the same component that is beneficial in moderate amounts. It is important to be aware of how it leaves us feeling. "Dosage" can make a difference in how it affects each person's mind and body because we are all biochemically unique. Sometimes chocolate acts to calm us, and sometimes it acts as a stimulant.

THE CHOCOLATE CURE?

Definition of Cure: *n. 1. a means of healing or restoring to health; remedy. 2. to relieve or rid. **Definition of Remedy:** n. 1. something, as a medicine, that cures or relieves a bodily disorder. 2. something that corrects or removes an evil or error. 3. to cure or relieve. 4. to put right; rectify.*

In the 1800s chocolate was purchased in apothecaries (drugstores).

Several hundred medicinal uses of cocoa have been discovered from as far back as 16th century European and Spanish manuscripts. Researchers are now studying some of these historical claims. Much of the recent research is about the antioxidant benefits. For example a year-long study completed in 2005 confirmed that the historical use of cocoa to treat diarrhea is a valid possibility. It was found that cocoa flavanoids can bind to and inhibit a protein that regulates fluid secretion in the small intestine.

Some migraine headache sufferers find chocolate can relieve symptoms, although one study showed a causal affect from chocolate in 30% of the participants. There is also anecdotal evidence that chocolate is helpful in eliminating or reducing some types of irritating coughs.

Cocoa...in a capsule? Some research scientists and pharmacists are considering adding cocoa to medicines to enhance their benefit. Also, a panel of scientists recently presented new data on the benefits of cocoa flavanols at the annual meeting of the American

Association for the Advancement of Science, which has led to consideration by pharmaceutical companies to synthesize the flavanol molecules in a laboratory for medical application.

Although cocoa contains opiate-like chemicals that produce endorphins in the brain, study participants who where given cocoa capsules, eliminating the feel of chocolate melting in their mouths, reported no "satisfying effect" at all. So while cocoa constituents might someday end up in our local pharmacy, it doesn't appear they'd ever replace the sensual experience of bars and desserts.

Whether scientists have a complete picture of all the health-enhancing benefits of chocolate remains to be seen. Given the increase in the world's consumption, chocolate lovers the world over aren't holding their breath waiting for more scientific evidence, but rather, are going ahead and "self medicating" with gusto!

THE DARKSIDE... BROUGHT INTO THE LIGHT!

CHOOSING CERTIFIED ORGANIC AND LOCAL

It's been estimated that more than 30 different pesticides are used in the growing of cocoa, one of the world's heaviest sprayed crops. One of these is a hormone disrupter called lindane, which has been linked to breast cancer. Lindane also poses serious health risks to cocoa farmers and workers.

For the health of the planet and our own health, choosing organic is always the wisest way to go. Why use pesticide and herbicide contaminated foods if we have the option to choose otherwise? 'Certified Organic' certification also ensures non-genetically modified ingredients are used as well, if you are choosing to avoid GM foods. I regularly compare prices and often find certain certified organic foods cost the same as, or sometimes even less than, their non-organic counterparts. Of course, where ever possible choose locally grown produce. It is the easiest on our environment, minimizing the pollution caused by transportation.

CHOOSING FAIR TRADE

Given the easy availability of chocolate in North America, and that it is a non-perishable product that can be easily transported, I assumed cocoa and chocolate were available world wide. I was shocked when I learned of the exploitation of young children and adults as slaves in the cocoa industry, most of whom don't even know what chocolate tastes like.

On the Ivory Coast, desperately poor cocoa farmers struggle to stay alive. Fifteen thousand children between the ages of 9 and 12 are working for minimal wages or as slaves for the chocolate industry. Reading of these horrors in Carol Off's book, **Bitter Chocolate** and the article, **"Is There Slavery in Your Chocolate?"** by John Robbins, will threaten the guilt-free attitude about chocolate I've attempted to build, but there IS something we can do.

To address the issue of inequity, fair trade certification began in 1988. It helps to empower farmers and farm workers to lift themselves out of poverty by investing in their farms and communities, by protecting the environment, and helping to develop business skills necessary for the underprivileged farmers to compete in the global marketplace.

Fortunately, there are now independent third-party certifiers of fair trade products, which participate in rigorous auditing practices to track products from farm to finished chocolate products and verify industry compliance with fair trade criteria.

It is my wish, my hope, my dream and my prayer that people will stop being exploited and everyone can enjoy the pleasures and nourishment of chocolate. We have the power to vote with our food dollars.

An excellent source of information on slavery in the chocolate industry, as well as a list of companies who use cocoa that has definitively NOT been produced with slave labor - **www.foodrevolution.org/slavery_chocolate.htm** The site also includes **"7 Things You Can Do"** to help stop slavery.

As well, purchase products displaying **ECO-TRADE** and **FAIR-TRADE** labels!

CHOCOLATE OF THE FUTURE?

Fortunate people around the globe will always enjoy the simple pleasure and indulgence of quality chocolate. The invigorating and uplifting affects of chocolate continue to provide endurance for the "superwomen and men" of today's busy world.

It appears there are no statistics showing how many people consciously use chocolate as a mood-enhancer and endurance tonic. While there is information about the natural chemicals responsible for these affects, I didn't find any surveys of the numbers of people who actually consume their favourite "morsels of ecstasy", as dependable food-drug therapy.

I imagine that more research will eventually enhance our understanding of what makes chocolate so remarkable. In the future, I wonder if other chemical benefits may be realized, as well as "dosage" awareness for health-enhancement. Can you imagine a day when doctor says to patient, "Take two dark chocolates and call me in the morning"? We can hope!

If advances are made in my lifetime, you'll find me reading that news, curled up in my coziest chair with my favourite mug of organic, fair trade, homemade, hot cocoa tonic!

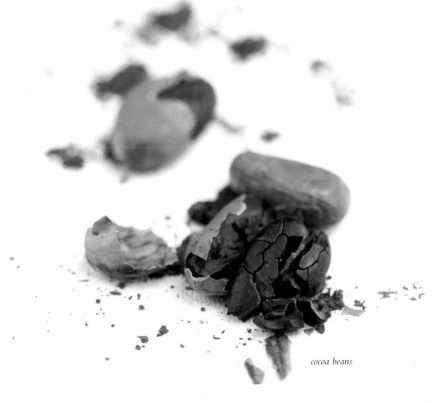

cocoa beans

PART 2

ALL ABOUT THE RADICAL NEW CHOCOLATE RECIPES

Why radical? **Health by Chocolate - Radical New Recipes**, dispells the myth that chocolate is just for dessert and has to be sugar-ladened and made with processed flour and high cholesterol fats to be mouth-watering, lip-smacking delicious. The recipes in this book are simple, easy and take only minutes to prepare.

They are suitable for anyone wanting to eat healthful, delicious snacks, meals, treats and desserts, and offer enzyme-rich, raw ingredients. All the recipes use whole food ingredients. (For the full description of "**What are Whole Foods?**" see **Part 1: THE LIGHTSIDE of CHOCOLATE**.)

As much as possible these recipes use fruits, fruit purees and nut-meats to sweeten. Maple syrup, honey and other natural sweeteners are also used. As well, they provide healthy fat, protein and complex carbohydrates from fresh nuts, nut-milks, tofu, whole grains and whole grain flours.

A number of the recipes are "raw", made directly in a blender or food processor without the need for heat, and some are done quickly on top of the stove in a pot with minimal ingredients and maximum flavour. Leftovers keep well refrigerated for days or even weeks, and pack well for travel.

Many of these recipes are also suitable for people with food or digestive challenges (eg. celiac disease, food sensitivities or IBS - Irritable Bowel Syndrome) and have symbols for easy identification.

Will using these recipes take the fun out of my chocolate indulgence? Absolutely not! These recipes are "guilt-free", healthy and nutritious. (Where and how you eat them is your choice, so they may not be "sin-free".) Seriously, the taste testers said over and over how great they felt after enjoying even the richest of these recipes. "These are awesome new twists on old favourites." All were taste-tested by a multi-aged team for "appeal-ability". Variations abound… so use these ideas to create new flavours from the base recipe and you'll never become bored.

Depending on your experience with whole food ingredients you may come across an unfamiliar ingredient, so an **INGREDIENT GLOSSARY** has been provided to help you. Learn about specific ingredients - where to purchase them, and how to use them, as well as some of their nutritional value. Once you become familiar with the ingredients and recipes, you will likely find they aren't so "radical" after all!

I decided to include only sweet recipes, so there are no savoury recipes in this book. However cocoa powder can also be included for added richness and flavour in savoury recipes such as chili, cornbread, pancakes, taco soup, mole, tortillas, and even pasta dishes. Cocoa, historically, was an important part of South American and other international cuisine, so go ahead and add a bit of cocoa goodness to your favourites.

All recipes were tested using imperial amounts; metric conversions are also provided. A food processor or blender (or hand wand or mixer) is required for some. Most recipes require minimal clean-up.

FROM CACAO BEAN TO CHOCOLATE BAR

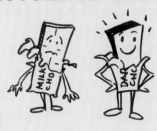

Up to 50 cacao beans fill each football shaped cacao pod, grown around the equator, on the cacao tree [Latin: theobroma cacao]. The shells are removed from the pods with sharp machetes, and the beans are cleaned and fermented for several days to improve their flavour. They are roasted from several minutes to several hours. The beans are crushed between large grinding stones or steel discs to form a dense liquid of peanut butter consistency, known as liquor. Despite the term, it contains no alcohol. Cacao liquor is compressed into bitter tasting (unsweetened) bars or separated into cacao butter and cacao mass. Cacao mass is then ground into powder. Cocoa powder is not completely fat free, retaining between 10-25% cocoa fat. Whole cacao beans and nibs (chopped pieces of beans) are about 50% fat. Dutch processed cocoa powder has been treated with an alkali during processing to produce a more mellow, darker coloured cocoa. This processing also removes much of the beneficial flavanols.

Cacao beans are not at all sweet, but bitter. If you nibble a raw cacao bean your mouth fills with a fullness that screams cocoa with a somewhat nutty flavour, but its not what our palates have been conditioned to anticipate. Raw **cacao nibs** are whole cacao beans that have been chopped into pieces and can be eaten alone as a snack, added to a nut and dried fruit trail mix or into recipes like some of those in this book. For most people some amount of sweetener is a must, but how much and what kind can make all the difference in whether the chocolate ends up healthful or harmful. Generally, the higher content of cocoa mass or liquor a chocolate bar contains, the lower the sugar content. Look for dairy-free dark chocolate bars with a high cocoa content (look for - mass, solids or liquor) of 70% or higher to enjoy the benefits of chocolate with less sugar. Also, not all sugars are created equally as you'll see in "THE LIGHTSIDE" part of this book, so look for the unrefined or less processed sugars. Milk chocolate typically contains much less cocoa content than dark chocolate, sometimes as low as 7%, because the milk fats and sugar ingredients make up the bulk. Inexpensive hydrogenated or highly processed fats are added to confectionery chocolate candy because it is cheaper for manufacturers to use as fillers, instead of pure cocoa butter.

Choosing a High Quality, Nutritious Chocolate Bar:
I considered including a "quality brand name chocolate bar comparison" (especially so I could justify all my chocolate bar sampling), however, I decided that would be unfair to you, because doing your own comparison sampling will be much more fun. Recently, there has been an influx of quality chocolate bars on the market. To know exactly what you're consuming check the ingredients list and label for the following:

LEAVE IT ON THE SHELF
- milk, milk fat, or lactose
- partially hydrogenated or hydrogenated oils
- Dutch processed or alkalized
- corn syrup, sugar
- confectionery chocolate
- artificial colours and flavours
- milk chocolate
- until you've read: **Bitter Chocolate** by Carol Off
or ...**www.foodrevolution.org/slavery_chocolate.htm**

ENHANCES OUR HEALTH
- 70% or higher dark chocolate
- dairy-free or vegan
- cocoa mass, liquor, solids, nibs
- cocoa butter
- cocoa powder
- pure vanilla and other flavour extracts
- grain or molasses sweetened
- cane juice or cane sugar
- certified organic ingredients
- fair trade symbols

THE HEALTHY CHOCOLATE KITCHEN GUIDE

Tips and know-how for easier CHOCOLATE PURCHASING, BAKING AND COOKING

Purchase quality baking/cooking chocolate in the form of chocolate chips, chunks, drops, bars or shavings with the same criteria used to pick out nutritious chocolate bars. You can find them in packages or in bulk bins, or in the baking or confectionary aisle of your grocery store, or health food market or chocolate shoppe (should you be so lucky!). Be sure to check ingredients and look for high cocoa content and low sugar content as much as possible. The names of sugars will vary and range from molasses to squeezed cane sugar. Watch for milk ingredients, even in "dark" chocolate. White "chocolate" is only cocoa butter mixed with sugar so should be avoided. Also, be aware of "decorator's" or "confectioner's" chocolate, as this is really only chocolate flavoured wax, used for coating fruit. For dipping fruit and a variety of other ingredients use a melted dark chocolate bar or chocolate with higher cocoa butter content such as "cooks" or "bakers" chocolate. Remember, whenever possible purchase fair trade and organic.

STORAGE - Always store chocolate in a cool, dry place, away from direct sunlight. Chocolate will 'bloom' (develop greyish-white streaks) due to temperature changes. The flavour is not affected however and it can still be melted for cooking.

RULES FOR MELTING CHOCOLATE

For dipping fruit or other ingredients use a melted dark chocolate bar or chocolate with higher cocoa butter content such as "cooks" or "bakers" chocolate.

▶ **NEVER ADD WATER** to melted chocolate, as it will ruin the glossy look and can create undesirable texture. If you need to thin it, add a touch of coconut or other oil. If you're dipping moist fruits, pat them dry with a towel before dipping.

▶ **MELT CHOCOLATE** directly in saucepan, double boiler, or in a glass bowl set over a pan filled with several inches of water over low heat (best way to avoid overheating or curdling). If you choose to microwave, use a glass bowl and cook on medium for one minute, stirring, then in 30 second bursts until melted. Use caution not to overheat it or the chocolate may scorch or burn.

▶ **CHOCOLATE SHOULD NEVER EXCEED 90°F (32°C)**. Remove from heat as soon as it melts or it will thicken or 'sieze'. If this happens you can whisk in a tablespoon full of oil, but it may have gone too far, in which case just make it into chocolate drops by adding your favourite ingredients (see RECIPES).

▶ **ALWAYS COOL LEFTOVER MELTED CHOCOLATE** before licking it to avoid burning your fingers or tongue. If you choose to avoid this rule, decide if the gain was worth the pain!

Of course, the easiest way to melt chocolate is to place it on your tongue ...and let it melt!

INGREDIENT GLOSSARY

DRIED & FRESH FRUITS are "nature's candy" and are loaded with antioxidant vitamins, minerals, fibres, enzymes, natural sweetness and flavours. Dried fruits are naturally concentrated in sugars as the water has been dried from them. They are usually available in bulk. Dried fruits that are brightly coloured usually have added sulphur and liquid sugars; non-sulphered fruits are not brightly coloured. Dried fruits and fruit purees are used successfully in these recipes, adding natural sweetness loaded with nutrients. Fresh fruits are used to enhance the flavour and nutrition of these healthy desserts and snacks. When you want chocolate with the flavour and goodness of fruits, you'll find a variety of choices in this book.

FROZEN BANANAS – High in potassium and B vitamins, I keep a large container in the freezer section of the fridge for easy access to these creamy delights. Whenever I notice bananas from my fruit bowl getting ripe, I top up my stock of frozen bananas in anticipation of making more summertime concoctions like ice cream, smoothies and other great treats. It's easy to place whole ripe bananas in your freezer with the skin still on. When you're ready to use them, soak them in a container of hot water for a minute or more, until you are able to slide the peel off the frozen flesh or run hot watter over the skin for at least a minute or more, peel back the skin and slide it off the banana flesh. Cut or break into chunks and place in food processor or blender. "It's as easy as banana pie!" (Alternately, you can also peel and cut bananas into chunks, and freeze on cookie sheets, which is more time consuming.) Always have a good supply of frozen bananas on hand, and you can make up a healthy delicious frozen or chilled treat in less time than it takes to run to the ice cream store.

MARIAH'S 'ON-THE-RUN' TRAIL MIX

1 handful	sunflower seeds
1 handful	pumpkin seeds
1 handful	broken or whole walnuts
	(or ½ cup pecans + ½ cup whole walnuts)
1 handful	dried blueberries, cherries or cranberries (or other dried fruit)
1 handful	dark, dairy-free chocolate chips (or ½ cup chips plus ½ cup cocoa nibs)

Mix together and store in an airtight container or ziplocked bag in the fridge for ultimate freshness. Adjust to suit your tastes. Quick and easy to make, this portable mix isn't just for hiking anymore. Enjoy it as a meal replacement when necessary, or a healthful snack anytime. Place in decorative glass jars for a thoughtful, nutritious gift.

NUTS & SEEDS – Purchase raw or dry roasted nuts and seeds. Because of their easily oxidized fats, most nuts and seeds should be purchased from the refrigerated section of grocery stores (you may have to look for a health food market), or from stores that have a good turnover, so nuts and seeds aren't sitting for very long periods without refrigeration. When you bring them home, store any bulk amounts in a fridge or freezer. Always avoid using any nuts/seeds or nut/seed products that have a rancid or sour smell. Flaxseeds and hempseeds are high sources of omega-3 fatty acids, beneficial for every cell in the body. The lignans in flaxseeds help to restore hormonal balance. Use them regularly and store them in refrigerated containers.

NUT & SEED BUTTER AND NUT FLOUR/MEAL – In these recipes you will find nut "butters" like hazelnut, almond, or cashew. These are made by grinding shelled, whole nuts or seeds, and are processed just like peanut butter. They can be found in most regular grocery or health food stores. Almond and hazelnut "flour", also called "meal", used in some of these recipes, is made from grinding raw whole nuts to a powder consistency. This can be done in a high powered blender or "Vitamix"…just don't grind too long or you'll end up with nut butter!

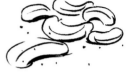

COCONUT OIL, COCONUT MILK AND COCONUT MEAT – The edible parts of the coconut provide important fatty acids, protein, fibre, minerals and, when raw, enzymes. Because of recent scientific research, coconut fat is making a comeback and is viewed as a healthful oil in appropriate amounts. Coconut oil, a good source of medium chain fatty acids, is a good choice for frying and baking, especially for those who've had their gallbladder removed. Some of the fatty acids are believed to be useful in reducing inflammation and candidiasis overgrowth. The antimicrobial properties of coconut oil are many. Coconut milk or cream (same product but sometimes labelled differently), is high in fat, and contain the same benefits as listed above for the oil. It is rich and creamy, and although the canned milk has no enzymes, it is wonderful for dessert making due to its unique flavour.

WHOLE GRAINS & WHOLE GRAIN FLOURS are always preferable to processed refined grains due to their superior nutritional components. Whole grains, when made into "white flour", even if labelled "organic" has much of the nutrition removed. Both the germ layer and the bran layer are stripped away, removing the beneficial fatty acids, vitamin E, fibre, much of the protein, B vitamins and minerals. "Enriched" flour simply means it's had a sprinkling of vitamins added back in. Whole grain flour should be purchased fresh, at stores that have good turnover, or from freshly ground flour you can make at home with a grain grinder. Small amounts of some grains can be ground fresh in quality blenders or "Vitamix" machines.

TOFU is made from soybeans, which contain phytoestrogens, believed to be helpful with menopausal symptoms such as hot flashes. There are several varieties and textures of tofu due to the coagulating factors that are used in the production of tofu. Unless you purchase it in a bulk pail, your tofu will have an expiration date. Fresh tofu (water packed or vacuum packed) should smell fresh, never sour. There should be no discoloration (pinkishness) on your tofu. A convenient way to always have tofu on hand is to purchase it in tetra paks. These "silken" varieties are great for dessert recipes like those in this book. "Lite" silken tofu is fat reduced and can be used to replace regular silken tofu. "Dessert" tofu has added sugar, and is not used in these recipes. Avoid "pressed tofu" for these recipes, as you want the creamier texture of the silken or fresh varieties. Pressed tofu and other firm versions are great for "meaty" recipes, whereas soft and medium, (or firm silken) usually work better for desserts. Commercial soy whipped topping (in spray cans) is also available.

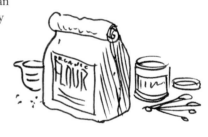

NATURAL SWEETENERS – Pure maple syrup is the sap of maple trees and provides manganese, zinc, calcium, potassium, and trace amounts of other minerals. Don't confuse "maple flavoured" syrup with pure maple syrup. Honey is the nectar of bees. Raw honey has antibacterial, antiviral and antifungal properties that have been said to be healing for a number of conditions. Blackstrap molasses is the residue from sugar cane production and is high in iron, calcium, copper, magnesium and potassium. Rich and delicious, be certain to use it in small quantities. "Table" or "cooking" molasses are not pure molasses but molasses mixed with other sweeteners. Agave nectar is the sugar of a cactus plant. Low on the glycemic index, it may be suitable for diabetics. Raw and natural sugars (eg. Sucanat™) are those that haven't been processed with high heat and have nutrients retained that aren't present after sugar is refined.

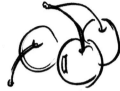

SPICES & HERBS can be used fresh or dried, and they add nutrition and flavour to desserts, as well as natural sweetness. For example, spices such as cinnamon, cardamom, coriander and star anise add sweetness. Use cinnamon liberally with these recipes as studies have shown its blood sugar balancing benefits. Ginger is warming and useful for nausea and better digestion. Mint is refreshing and lightens up a richer dessert. Cacao nibs (chopped pieces of raw dried cocoa beans) have a delicious chocolate flavour and a nutty, crunchy texture that can be added to cookies and other recipes, or eaten alone or with fruits and nuts. Carob powder is sometimes used as a cocoa powder substitute. It contains some similar nutrients, but does not contain the flavanoids or phytochemicals found in cocoa bean. In some of these and other recipes it can partially or completely replace the cocoa powder.

AGAR, KUZU & ARROWROOT are natural thickeners. Agar (available in bars, flakes and powder) is derived from sea vegetable and is used as a vegetarian "gelatin". Kuzu is the starch from the root of the wild kuzu plant and is dissolved in liquid and simmered to thicken sauces. It is said to have digestive benefits. Arrowroot, the most economical thickener, comes from a native American plant.

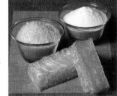

Agar

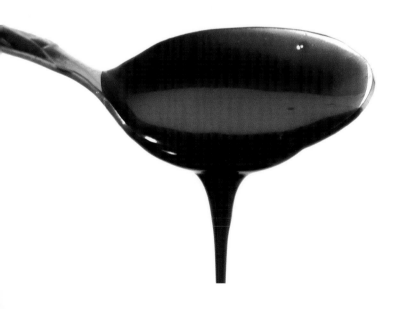

HEALTH BY CHOCOLATE
RADICAL NEW RECIPES

From temptation...to sensation...to salvation.
Turn up your taste buds, tune up your heart,
transform your mind and tease your libido
with these delightful healthy chocolate recipes!

SECTION #4 – Cakes & Cookies, Bars & Bonbons – pg. 75

In response to the growing numbers of people who have food allergies or food sensitivities, the following symbols have been included in each recipe to allow for easy identification. ALL recipes in HEALTH by CHOCOLATE are Egg and Dairy Free.

SYMBOLS

The symbols on each recipe page identify the following:

The "V" on the end means Variation (eg. GFV =gluten free variation)

GF = gluten free
WF = wheat free
NF = nut free
SF = soy free
RW = raw (or mostly raw food) ingredients

Note: Always check the ingredient list of melting chocolate: (chocolate chips, bars, drops, chunked, or shaved chocolate) for soy lecithin (soy), or nut oils (nuts), or grain sweeteners (gluten), if you have a severe allergy or celiac disease.

Caution: Always use your own judgement when preparing these recipes if allergies are a concern. Symbols are provided as a guideline for easy access, and while great care was taken with the symbol labeling, the author is not responsible for any error that may have occurred. Some of these recipes contain nuts, which can be potential allergens. Advise people to whom you serve them that they contain nuts, as they may be unsuspecting due to the creamy nature of some of the recipes.

"…the primary fat in chocolate is stearic acid, and as far as fats go, it's not bad. It is a saturated vegetable fat, but unlike most saturated animal fats, stearic acid acts in the body much like the monounsaturated fat in olive oil. Monounsaturates have a neutral effect on cholesterol."

from **Health by Chocolate** *foreword*
by John Robbins

SECTION #1 CHOCOLATE TONICS & BEVERAGES, SMOOTHIES & ICY TREATS

Calming Chocolate
Tonic
pg. 37

Creamy Cashew
Chocolate Milk
pg. 39

Malted Calci-yum
Rich Chocolate Smoothie
pg. 41

Nutty Chocolate
Banana Buds
pg. 43

Natural Ice
Cream
pg. 45

Chocolate Cherry
Fountain Drink
pg. 47

Knickerbocker
Glory Parfait
pg. 49

DID YOU KNOW?

Coconut milk is easily digested by people who have had their gall bladder removed because it doesn't require bile to break it down.

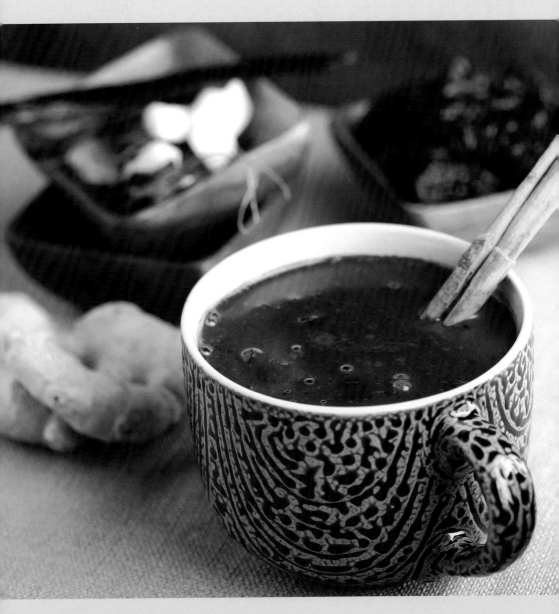

Tester Comments

"Rich, creamy and delicious, I loved all the variations."

"Warm and soothing."

"Heavenly!"

CALMING CHOCOLATE TONIC

This rich, creamy, hot chocolate "tonic" pays homage to the Aztecs who first consumed cacao as a beverage. I love the idea of this warm delicious drink as a "therapeutic" beverage. Certainly it warms the heart as well as the body, especially if you sip it with someone you adore.

Makes: 2-4 servings

15 oz can (425 ml)	**coconut milk**
2 Tbsp (30 ml)	**cocoa powder**
¼ cup (60 ml)	**pure maple syrup, pure honey or dry sweetener**
pinch	**salt**

Optional ingredients:

1 tsp (5 ml)	**pure vanilla extract or 1 vanilla bean**
4 slices	**fresh ginger root**
	pinch chili powder
½ tsp (2 ml)	**ground cinnamon or 1 cinnamon stick**
½ tsp (2 ml)	**ground cardamom or coriander powder**
1 tsp (5 ml)	**instant coffee** (or chai tea bag)

Whisk together the coconut milk, cocoa, salt and sweetener and any optional ingredients, in a small pan over medium heat until steaming. Pour into your favourite mug and sip slowly and mindfully, enjoying every mouthful of pure pleasure.

(Remove ginger root, teabag or cinnamon stick before serving.)

VARIATION

▸ To reduce fat content, other nut milks <u>or</u> soymilk can replace all or some coconut milk, but coconut is the smoothest, richest and most delicious.

▸ Optional Treat for Special Occasions: Top with SILKY WHIPPED CREAMY TOPPING - See Section 3 - either homemade or purchased, and sprinkle with cinnamon or cocoa powder!

The Mayas revered cocoa and used it as a special drink for marriage and other ceremonies.

Cashews have the lowest fat content of the nut family, and are a good source of many minerals and B vitamins. They are good for muscles and nerves. They spoil quickly, so keep refrigerated.

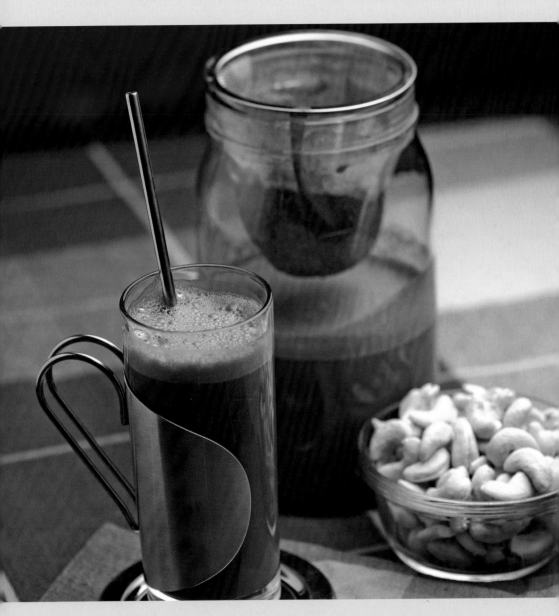

Tester Comments

"So easy to make and so refreshing."
"The espresso variation is yummy."
"Scrumptious, my favourite. Tastes very much like a frosty."

CREAMY CASHEW CHOCOLATE MILK

More nutritious than commercially pasteurized milks and beverages; nut milks retain their enzymes providing "sparkplug energy". This family favourite is full of chocolatey richness. You can strain the cashew bits from this recipe or leave them in, creating a funky drink that reminds me of a "bubble tea" concept.

Makes: 3-4 servings

1 cup (250 ml)	**raw cashews**
4 Tbsp (60 ml)	**maple syrup**
3 Tbsp (45 ml)	**cocoa powder**
2½ cups (625 ml)	**water** (1 + 1½ cups)

Place cashews, syrup and cocoa powder in a tall glass jar with approximately 1 cup water. Blend well with a hand blender until smooth and creamy, or put ingredients in a blender and process until smooth and creamy.

Add the remaining water and blend well.

Note: If you wish to strain the cashew bits, pour milk through a straining bag or cheesecloth-lined strainer (unnecessary if you like a bit of chewiness in the bottom of your glass).

Serve over ice cubes or refrigerate before serving. Will keep for 2-3 days.

VARIATION

▸ CREAMY CASHEW CHOCOLATE FROSTY
Using the recipe above add 2 cups (500 ml) ice cubes or for a creamier version, use 2 cups (500 ml) of frozen banana instead of, or as well as, ice cubes. Blend until frosty.

▸ ESPRESSO
Add 1 tsp (5 ml) ground instant coffee granules.

▸ CHOCOLATE CHAI
Mix in equal quantities with chai concentrate or sweetened spicy chai tea.

Chocolate is cheaper than therapy, and you don't need an appointment.

Blackstrap molasses and tahini are high in calcium and other important minerals for bone building. Essential fatty acids in hemp seeds are also crucial bone building nutrients. Cocoa also contains calcium, magnesium, iron, potassium and trace minerals…so load up on this delicious beverage!

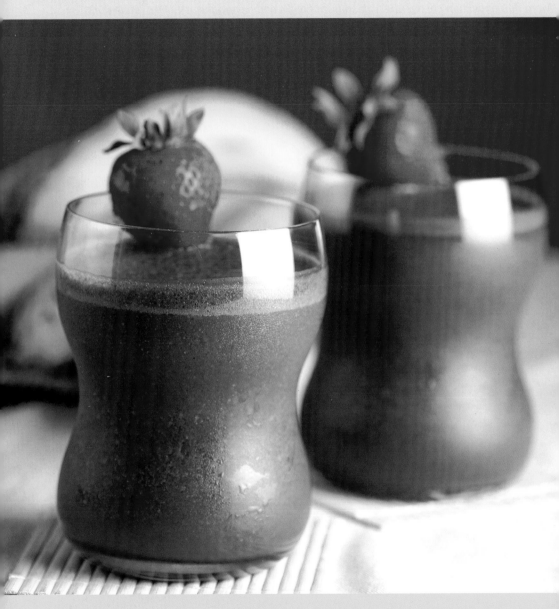

Tester Comments

"I really love this bone building smoothy that is so delicious."
"Easy to drink, enjoy and run!"
"I make it a regular smoothie, so I don't have to take calcium supplements."

MALTED CALCI-YUM RICH CHOCOLATE SMOOTHIE

Calcium isn't just for bone building. It is also essential for heart health and the nervous system. This smoothie is enjoyed by anyone who loves the creamy, rich blend of malted flavours.

Makes: 3-4 servings

4	**large frozen bananas**
4	**ice cubes (or 8 if bananas aren't frozen)**
2½ cups (625 ml)	**cold water** (or unsweetened, calcium-fortified soy beverage)
3 Tbsp (45 ml)	**cocoa powder**
2 Tbsp (30 ml)	**tahini (sesame butter)**
1 Tbsp (15 ml)	**hulled hemp seeds**
2 Tbsp (30 ml)	**pure maple syrup**
2 tsp (10 ml)	**blackstrap molasses**

Blend all ingredients, except molasses, in a blender.

Add molasses last by drizzling it in while the blender is running to prevent it from sinking to the bottom.

Blend until smooth and creamy.

VARIATION

► Need a little more caffeine with your calcium? Add 1 tsp instant coffee dissolved in 1 Tbsp boiling water for an Espresso Chocolate Malted variation.

There is a theory that chocolate slows down the aging process...it may not be true, but do you really want to take a chance?!

Bananas are high in potassium, but they also are a source of vitamin B6, folic acid, vitamin C, riboflavin and magnesium.
Maybe a "banana-a-day" keeps the doctor away too.

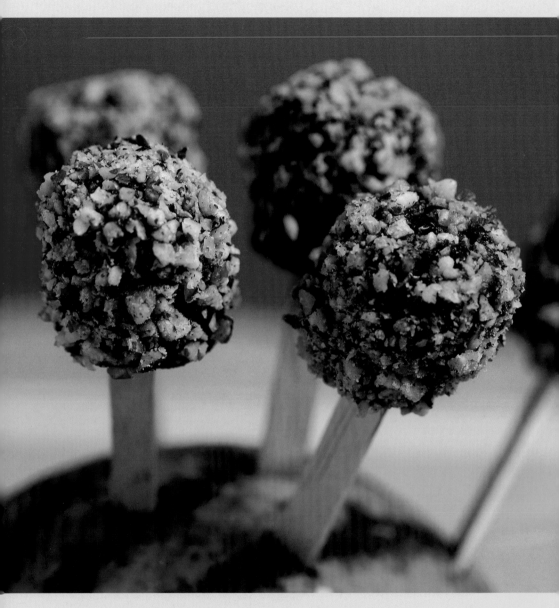

Tester Comments

"I made these for my husband's staff. They didn't make it to the office, but disappeared from the freezer in some mysterious and completely unexplained fashion. However, the thief was kind enough to leave the empty pan behind in the freezer - presumably for future use."
"Sweet cold banana and nutty chocolate are the best combination ever!"

NUTTY CHOCOLATE BANANA BUDS

These bite size treats are a creamy, crunchy, cool delight. Preparation in advance is easy and takes only minutes. Banana buds make a great end to a meal, or a light snack anytime.

Makes: 10 - 12 buds

2	ripe medium-large bananas
10 -12	wooden or plastic popsicle sticks
½ **cup** (125 ml)	hazelnuts or pecans, chopped, or hulled hemp seeds or cocoa nibs
¾ **cup** (175 ml)	dark chocolate chips or melting chocolate

Prepare at least one hour in advance of serving.

Line a baking sheet or a freezer-safe flat plate with plastic wrap or parchment paper. Peel and cut bananas into 1" pieces. Pierce each banana bud with a popsicle stick. Place each banana bud, stick side up, on the prepared sheet and place in freezer for 30-45 minutes or more.

Chop nuts with a knife or in a food processor. Place in a shallow dish and set aside.

Melt chocolate - See rules in section ABOUT RECIPES.

Remove 3 or 4 banana buds from freezer at a time and roll each bud in melted chocolate until covered. Roll in nuts. Repeat for each bud. Place the coated buds back on sheet in freezer until chocolate sets.

VARIATION

▶ NUT-FREE VARIATION - replace nuts with hulled hemp seeds.

▶ Replace chocolate chips with your favourite flavoured dark chocolate bar.

Note: You can purchase popsicle sticks at Dollar or Craft Stores.

There is more to life than chocolate, but not right now.

Cocoa nibs are chopped pieces of the raw cocoa bean and have a nutty texture.
Try sprinkling a few over your next "Natural Sundae" treat.

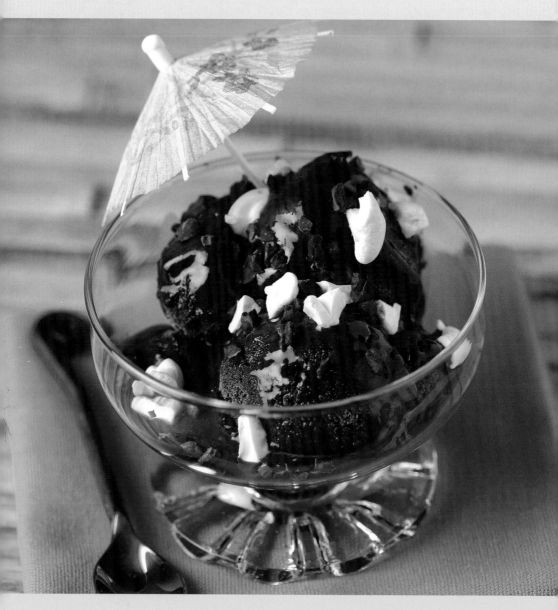

Tester Comments

"Ice cream without guilt…I can eat as much as I want and not feel like I'm on a sugar high."
"I love the Sundae with the syrup…and the nibs are pretty interesting too."

NATURAL ICE CREAM

Yummy! You won't miss the "after-effects" of commercial ice cream when you enjoy this light delicious chocolatey treat…summertime or anytime!

Makes: 2 servings

2	large frozen bananas
2 Tbsp (30 ml)	honey, maple syrup or agave nectar
1 tsp (5 ml)	vanilla
3-4 Tbsp (45-60 ml)	cocoa powder

Optional Additions:

¼ cup (60 ml)	chopped nuts
1 Tbsp (15 ml)	cocoa nibs
½-1 cup	chopped fruit

Remove the skins of frozen bananas by soaking in a container of hot tap water, running under hot water for about 2 minutes and peel. Cut or break each banana into 5-6 sections and process them in a food processor with the 'S' blade until creamy.

Add sweetener, vanilla and cocoa powder to food processor. Process until creamy, several minutes if necessary, to blend ingredients well (you're aiming for the consistency of soft ice cream).

Serve immediately "as is" for "soft" ice cream or place in the freezer for 20-30 minutes for "harder" ice cream or if not serving immediately.

Ice cream will store for several days in a sealed container in the freezer. Texture may change to more of a sorbet type texture, depending on the ripeness of the bananas.

Note: If you own a homogenizer juicer (eg. Champion), you can make easy creamy ice cream, by feeding the ingredients through the feeder tube with the blank inserted instead of the screen.

VARIATION

▶ NATURAL ICE CREAM SUNDAE
Make delicious "sundaes" by drizzling SIMPLE CHOCOLATE SYRUP - Section 3 over ice cream, and top with chopped nuts, cocoa nibs, coconut flakes, fruit sauce, or fresh fruit and WHIPPED CREAMY TOPPING - Section 3.

In 1660 ladies of the court began drinking cocoa and when they were told it was an aphrodisiac, demand for cocoa skyrocketed in France.

DID YOU KNOW?

Black cherry juice is traditionally used for "gouty" arthritis.

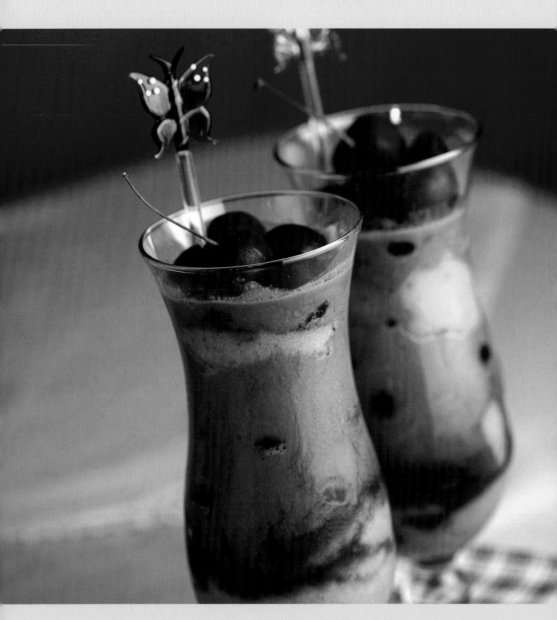

Tester Comments

"Wow, cherries and chocolate…my favourite combination in one delicious drink…I could make this a habit."

CHOCOLATE CHERRY FOUNTAIN DRINK

Inspired by Food TV personality and author Rachel Ray, whom I understand began her cooking career as a fountain girl, this version uses healthful guilt-free ingredients.

Makes: 4 servings

1 cup (250 ml)	**pitted cherries, chopped** (put 4 whole cherries aside)
4	**large frozen bananas** (or 4 servings of NATURAL ICE CREAM - Section 1)
1 cup (250 ml)	**pure cherry juice**
8 Tbsp (120 ml)	**CASHEW CHOCOLATE MILK - Section 1**

Note:

▶ Use fresh, frozen or reconstituted dried cherries.

▶ You can purchase organic soy whipped cream in a spray bottle, for the traditional spiral topped look.

VARIATION

▶ Large dollops SILKY WHIPPED CREAMY TOPPING - Section 3

▶ ½ cup (125 ml) plain soda water.

▶ Place a squirt of SIMPLE CHOCOLATE SYRUP in each glass - Section 3

Pit cherries and cut into halves or quarters.

Use either Chocolate NATURAL ICE CREAM, or frozen bananas:

Remove the skins of frozen bananas by soaking in a container of hot tap water, running under hot water for about 2 minutes and peel. Cut or break each banana into 5-6 sections and process them in a food processor with the 'S' blade until creamy.

Process until creamy, several minutes if necessary (you're aiming for the consistency of soft ice cream).

Place a large scoop into each of 4 parfait or deep glasses. Add to each glass a layer each of cherries, cherry juice and CREAMY CASHEW CHOCOLATE MILK.

Place a spoon in each glass for serving. Decorate each with a whole cherry.

Seven days without chocolate makes one weak.

DID YOU KNOW?

Cocoa beans were often used as currency in historical times…I guess money really does grow on trees!

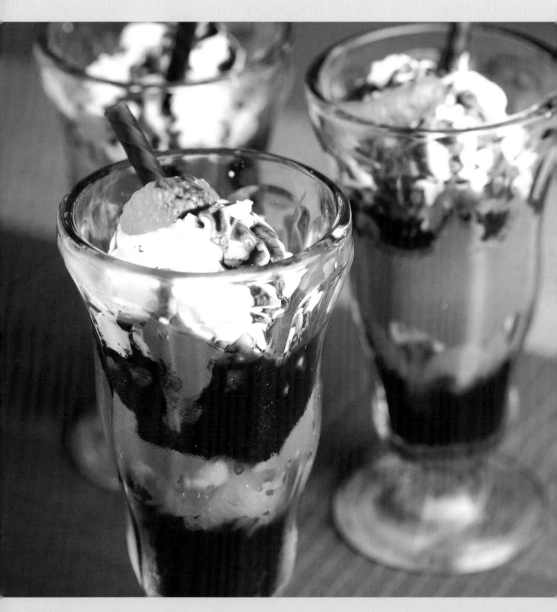

Tester Comments

"Wow! This was a big hit with everyone, young and old."
"Amazing! This is the best parfait I've ever had in my life."
"This is so much fun."

KNICKERBOCKER GLORY PARFAIT

My British friend introduced me to this treat, which can be made in a variety of ways. In the first Harry Potter book, cousin Dudley had a tantrum at the zoo because his knickerbocker glory wasn't big enough, so Harry became the pleased recipient.

Makes: 4-6 servings depending on size

Easy Ice Cream:

2	**large frozen bananas**
2 Tbsp (30 ml)	**honey, maple syrup or agave nectar**
1 tsp (5 ml)	**vanilla**
3-4 Tbsp (45-60 ml)	**cocoa powder**

Parfait ingredients:

2 cups (500 ml)	**fruit puree or chopped fruit**
⅓ cup (75 ml)	**chopped nuts**

Choices: See SECTIONS…
#3 - SIMPLE CHOCOLATE SYRUP
#2 - CHOCOLATE MOUSSE
#2 - CHOCOLATE AVOCADO CUSTARD
#2 - INSTANT CHOCOLATE PUDDING
#3 - SILKY WHIPPED CREAMY TOPPING

CHOCOLATE ICE CREAM:

Remove the skins of frozen bananas by soaking in a container of hot tap water, running under hot water for about 2 minutes and peel. Cut or break each banana into 5-6 sections and process them in a food processor with the 'S' blade until creamy.

Add sweetener, vanilla and cocoa powder to food processor. Process until creamy, several minutes if necessary, to blend ingredients well (you're aiming for the consistency of soft ice cream). Use immediately or place in freezer.

TO MAKE PARFAIT:

Layer parfait glasses from bottom to top, in the order you choose, with as many choices as you desire, and drizzle with SIMPLE CHOCOLATE SYRUP:

- ice cream
- mousse, custard or pudding
- fruit puree or chopped fruit
- chopped nuts
- whipped cream

Chocolate: here today…gone today!

"...chocolate also boosts brain levels of serotonin. Women typically have lower serotonin levels during PMS and menstruation, which may be one reason women typically experience stronger cravings for chocolate than men. People suffering from depression so characteristically have lower serotonin levels that an entire class of anti-depressive medications called serotonin uptake inhibitors (including Prozac, Paxil, and Zoloft) have been developed that raise brain levels of serotonin."

*from **Health by Chocolate** foreword*
by John Robbins

SECTION #2
PUDDINGS & PIES, SAUCES & SPREADS

Instant Chocolate
Pudding or Pie Filling
pg. 53

Quick Creamy Chocolate
Avocado Custard
pg. 55

Rich Chocolate
Mousse
pg. 57

Nutty-Ella Chocolate
Spread
pg. 59

Orange Chocolate
Meltdown Fondue
or Dipping Sauce
pg. 61

Pineapple Banana
Pecan Divinity
pg. 63

Baked Strawberry
Puddles
pg. 65

Raspberry Crème
Cups
pg. 67

Passion in a Pan
pg. 69

DID YOU KNOW?

Carob is a ground pod that some use as a chocolate substitute because it does not contain caffeine. It may have a similar texture and color, but the flavour is different and it does not have the same phytochemicals.

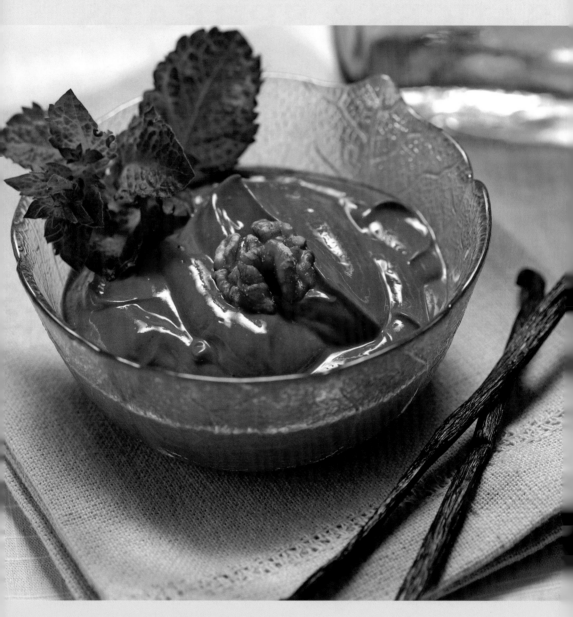

Tester Comments

" Yummy…so quick and easy to make."

INSTANT CHOCOLATE PUDDING OR PIE FILLING

So simple and easy to make, you can even teach young children to make this low-fat recipe. Have fun being creative with additional flavours.

Makes: 4-6 servings of pudding or filling for two pies

1-12 oz (349 g)	**pkg soft or medium silken tofu**
⅓-½ cup (75-125 ml)	**pure maple syrup** (or 6-8 large moist dates, pitted)
⅓ cup (75 ml)	**dark cocoa or carob powder**
1-2 tsp (5-10 ml)	**pure vanilla extract**
pinch	**salt**

Optional:

1-2 Tbsp (15-30 ml)	**cashew or almond butter**
¼ cup (60 ml)	**chopped pecans or walnuts to be sprinkled on top**
2 tsp (10 ml)	**ground cinnamon**
1 tsp (5 ml)	**ground cardamom**
1 tsp (5 ml)	**mint extract**

Note: This recipe can be used as a pie filling for your favourite whole grain pie crust, (or use CHOCOLATE GINGER PECAN PIE mixture - Section 4 - to make two unbaked crusts).

If using dates, soak them in hot water for several minutes to soften.

Place all ingredients in a blender or food processor and blend several minutes until smooth and creamy.

Pour into individual serving bowls.

Serve immediately or chill in fridge until serving time.

VARIATION

▶ Replace some or all cocoa powder with carob powder.

Is a balanced diet chocolate in both hands?

DID YOU KNOW?

Avocados are higher in potassium than bananas. They are a good source of vitamin E, K, B6, C, copper, folate, and lutein. Avocados have healthy fatty acids that studies have shown can help to protect against prostate and breast cancers, and heart disease.

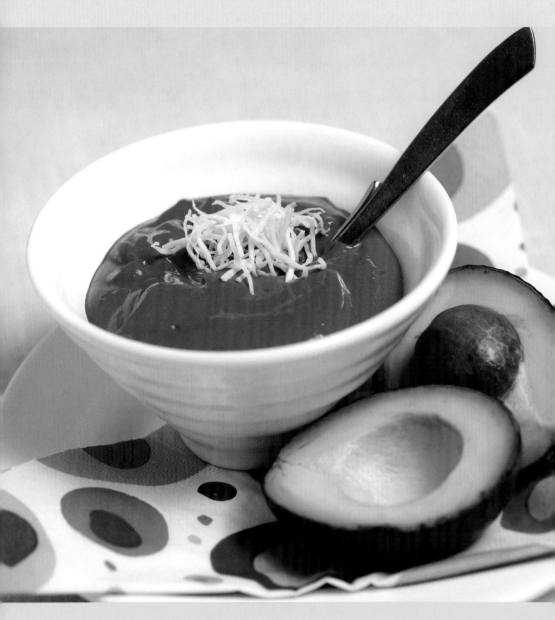

Tester Comments

"I just thought this was terrific."
"I can't believe there's avocado in this. It's hard to believe that something this delicious could be so healthy."

QUICK CREAMY CHOCOLATE AVOCADO CUSTARD

This non-dairy, non-soy pudding is as creamy and decadent as traditional versions.

Makes: approximately 6 servings

½ **cup** (125 ml)	**dates,** (soaked for 5-10 minutes in hot water and drained)
1¾ - 2 cups (395-500 ml)	**mashed avocado** (2-4 avocados depending on size)
½ **cup** (125 ml)	**cocoa powder**
2 Tbsp (30 ml)	**vanilla**
1 tsp (5 ml)	**ground cinnamon** (optional)
¼ tsp (1 ml)	**sea salt**
½ **cup** (125 ml)	**maple syrup**

In a food processor, using the 'S' blade, blend all ingredients for several minutes until creamy. If you find the consistency is too thick, drizzle in a spoonful of water at a time until desired consistency is reached.

Divide among individual serving dishes and chill.

Optional: Decorate with a dollop of SILKY WHIPPED CREAMY TOPPING - Section 3, if desired. Garnish with any of the following; mint leaves, strawberries, raspberries, coconut, chopped nuts.

VARIATION

▶ CREAMY BANANA CHOCOLATE PUDDING
  Replace avocados with ripe banana.

▶ Replace dates, cocoa and syrup with 1¼ cups (310 ml) dark chocolate chips, melted.

▶ Use for frosting a cake or cupcakes.

If only writers' blocks were made of chocolate.

While coconut milk is high in fat, in appropriate quantities it is healthful and has many beneficial properties that include fighting viral, bacterial, fungal and yeast infections. It is thought to boost metabolism and assist in weight loss. Serve it up with a simple meal of fibre filled lentils or beans and a large veggie salad, and there will be nothing to feel guilty about!

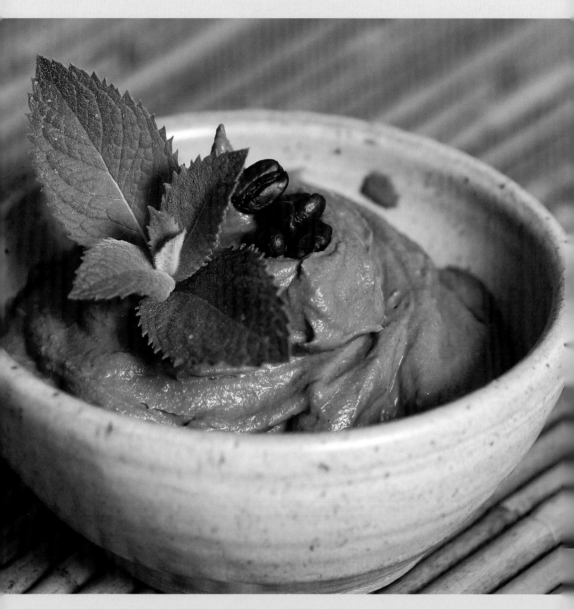

Tester Comments

"This is the most decadent mousse I've ever tasted…It really is 'to live for'."
"Incredibly delicious, everyone loved it."
"The best mousse I've EVER tasted! I like the hint of cinnamon."
"This has become my 'menopausal mousse'…my favourite comfort food."

RICH CHOCOLATE MOUSSE

Smooth, creamy and delicious…this exquisite mousse melts in your mouth.

Makes: 6 servings

2 - 14 oz (400 ml) **cans**	**coconut milk**
1 Tbsp (23 ml) **(or 3 Tbsp** (45 ml)	**agar powder** **agar flakes)**
1 cup (250 ml)	**raw sugar** (see note)
½ cup (125 ml)	**unsweetened cocoa powder**
1 tsp (5 ml)	**pure vanilla extract**
½ -1 tsp (5 ml)	**ground cinnamon**
⅛ tsp (0.5 ml)	**salt**
¾ cup (175 ml)	**cold water**
2 Tbsp (60 ml)	**arrowroot powder or kuzu powder or cornstarch**

Note: See ingredient glossary for agar and arrowroot powder.

VARIATION

▸ ESPRESSO MOUSSE: Add 2 Tbsp (30 ml) cold espresso or 1 tsp (5 ml) instant coffee granules dissolved in 2 Tbsp (30 ml) hot water.

▸ MOCHA BREAKFAST PARFAIT: Layer ESPRESSO MOUSSE variation with your favourite granola and slices of banana in a bowl or glass.

Note: I usually use Sucanat™ sugar for this recipe but you can replace the sugar with 1 cup maple syrup and increase agar to 2 Tbsp powder or 4 Tbsp flakes.

In a large saucepan, combine coconut milk and agar. Add sugar, cocoa, vanilla, cinnamon and salt.

Simmer for 3-5 minutes until agar has completely dissolved (check by dipping a spoon into mixture).

In a small bowl, whisk together the cold water and arrowroot until smooth. Pour into the saucepan, whisking for approximately 1 minute, until mixture thickens.

Cool at room temperature or in the fridge.

Pour cooled mixture into food processor and puree until creamy. Serve chilled in individual cups or parfait glasses.

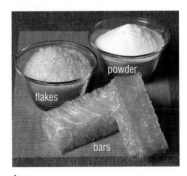

Agar

Forget love…I'd rather fall in chocolate!

While prunes are not the highest fruit source of dietary fibre, they do have phytochemicals that assist the body "to get things moving".

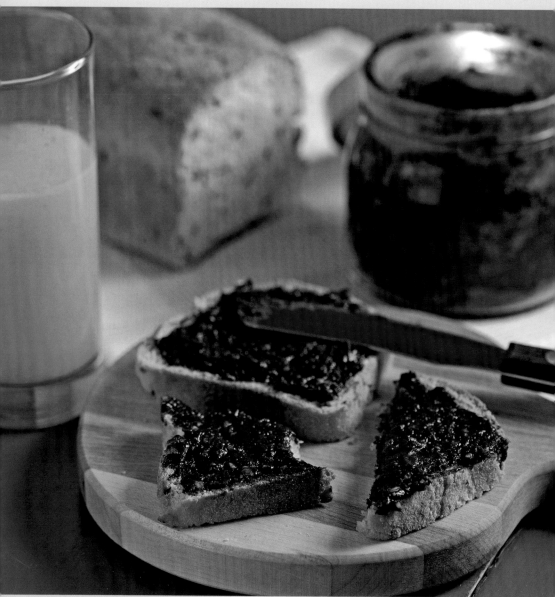

Tester Comments

"This is a great and novel way to get my morning prunes."
"Really? There's prunes in this…amazing."

NUTTY-ELLA CHOCOLATE SPREAD

Try it, you'll like it! No one will ever suspect it's good for them and it makes a popular toast spread.

Makes: 2½ cups

1 cup (250 ml)		**pitted prunes**
½ cup (125 ml)		**cocoa or carob powder**
½ cup (125 ml)		**honey**
1 tsp (5 ml)		**ground cinnamon**
2 tsp (10 ml)		**vanilla**
¼ cup (60 ml)		**hazelnut butter**
¼ cup (60 ml)		**chopped hazelnuts or hazelnut meal flour**

Note: You can purchase commercially prepared, finely ground hazelnuts as "flour" or "meal", or chop nuts in a food processor.

Put prunes and enough water to cover them, in a saucepan with a lid. Simmer covered until prunes are soft (usually 3-5 minutes). Drain water.

In a food processor add drained prunes and the rest of the ingredients and process until mixed.

Transfer to a container to cool.

Spread on warm toast or crackers.

VARIATION

▶ Replace hazelnut butter with peanut butter.

▶ Replace chopped hazelnuts with pecans or walnuts.

Put "eat chocolate" at the top of your list of things to do today. That way, at least you'll get one thing done.

DID YOU KNOW?

Tofu, made from soybeans and coagulated with minerals, is available in many forms: soft, medium, firm and extra firm, as well as pressed, marinated and smoked flavours. Versatile and easy to use, keep the unrefrigerated, tetra pak, silken version on hand in your cupboard and you'll have a ready source.

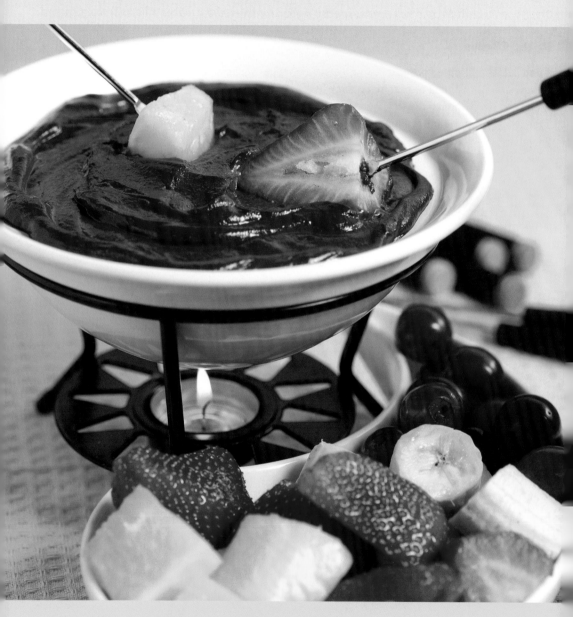

Tester Comments

"What a great and easy entertaining idea…everyone loved it."
"I love the orange flavour and the creamy texture."

ORANGE CHOCOLATE MELTDOWN
FONDUE OR DIPPING SAUCE

If you love the combination of chocolate and orange, you'll love this creamy dip warmed or chilled. Use your imagination for different "dippers".

Makes: 4-6 servings

12 oz (349 g)	**silken tofu** (soft or medium)
¼ cup (60 ml)	**orange juice concentrate**
1 tsp (5 ml)	**ground cinnamon** (optional)
1 cup (250 ml)	**chocolate chips**

Suggested Dippers:
▸ **pineapple wedges**
▸ **banana slices**
▸ **strawberries**
▸ **orange slices**
▸ **apples slices**
▸ **dried dates, apricots, or figs**
▸ **day old wholegrain bread, cake or muffins, cut into chunks**

Reluctant Veggie Eaters?
▸ **cauliflower or broccoli florets**
  (raw or lightly steamed)
▸ **celery sticks**

Anything goes if it means more veggies!

Blend tofu, juice concentrate, and cinnamon with a blender or hand blender.

Melt chocolate - See rules in section ABOUT RECIPES.

Scrape into tofu mixture and blend again until incorporated.

For Fondue: scrape mixture into fondue dish to warm, or warm first in the same saucepan as the chips were melted.

For Dipping Sauce: scrape into a serving bowl and serve immediately or chill in fridge before serving.

VARIATION

▸ CAKE FROSTING
Increase chocolate chips to 1½ cups (375 ml).
Chill and spread on cake or cupcakes.

If at first you don't succeed...
have a chocolate.

DID YOU KNOW?

Pineapple is high in bromelain which helps to reduce inflammation and is a digestive aid.

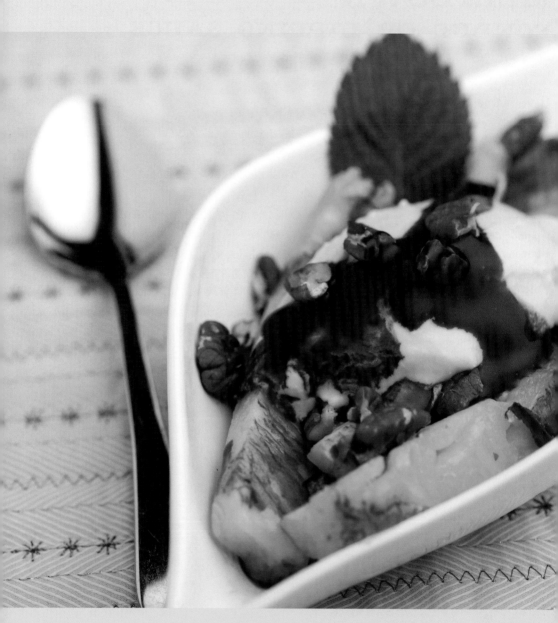

Tester Comments

"This really is divine, everyone loved it. I've been eating it on my pancakes every morning."

PINEAPPLE BANANA PECAN DIVINITY

The natural sweetness and flavours are enhanced when the fruits and nuts are warmed.

Makes: 4 servings

½ cup	**SIMPLE CHOCOLATE SYRUP - Section 3**
1 Tbsp (15 ml)	**coconut oil**
half	**fresh pineapple**
2	**bananas, peeled** (use firm ripe bananas)
½ cup (125 ml)	**pecans, chopped**
¼ cup (60 ml)	**cocoa nibs (optional)**

VARIATION

▶ For an even richer dessert, top with a dollop of SILKY WHIPPED CREAMY TOPPING - Section 3, CASHEW COCONUT CREAM - Section 3, ORANGE CHOCOLATE MELTDOWN DIPPING SAUCE - Section 2, or soy vanilla ice cream.

▶ This recipe also makes a great crepe filling.

Grease a casserole or baking dish with coconut oil.

Core a fresh pineapple and slice into "fingers". Slice bananas in half cross-wise. Then slice each half lengthwise into four finger-like pieces (8 pieces for each banana).

Place the fruit in the baking dish and sprinkle the pecans evenly over top.

Broil 6" from the heat for about 3-4 minutes, or in toaster oven until nuts are toasted and fruits are softened (2-3 minutes).

Make a batch of SIMPLE CHOCOLATE SYRUP - Section 3.

Drizzle with warm chocolate syrup or any other favourite chocolate topping. Sprinkle with cocoa, cocoa nibs or ground cinnamon.

Seen on T-shirt : EMERGENCY ALERT - If wearer of this shirt is found vacant, listless, or depressed, ADMINISTER CHOCOLATE IMMEDIATELY.

DID YOU KNOW?

The Aztecs associated cocoa with the goddess of fertility (Xochiquetzal), and the spicy cocoa drink seasoned with vanilla, chili pepper and other spices, was called Xocoatl.

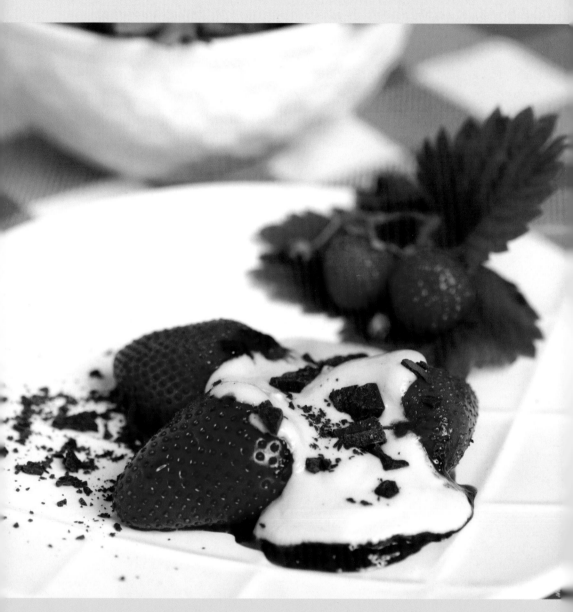

Tester Comments

"I liked the fact that the sauce was not too rich."
"I like the uniqueness and the surprise of the chocolate."
"At first glance this recipe seemed a little daunting, but my mom and I made it together and it really didn't take very long and turned out to be fun."

BAKED STRAWBERRY PUDDLES

The puddle of chocolate that oozes out of the berries becomes a delightful unexpected treat. Friends and family will enjoy the elegant simplicity of this dessert.

Makes: 4 servings

12	large whole strawberries
½ cup (125 ml)	dark chocolate chips or shaved chocolate bar
½ cup (125 ml)	orange juice
2 tsp (10 ml)	grated ginger root
1 cup (250 ml)	**SILKY CREAMY WHIPPED TOPPING - Section 3**

VARIATION

▶ Omit ginger, should you desire.

Preheat oven or toaster oven to 350°F.

Rinse berries. Core the inside of each whole berry with a grapefruit spoon or small sharp knife, removing stem at the same time.

Pour orange juice into a baking pan. Grate the ginger into the pan and stir. Fill each berry with chocolate, stuffing each one as much as possible. Place each berry upside down or on its side.

Bake for approximately 5-7 minutes until chocolate has melted. Remove from oven and place 3 berries on each individual serving plate.

Top with a dollop of SILKY WHIPPED CREAMY TOPPING

Optional: Sprinkle each serving with cinnamon or cocoa powder for extra garnish or decorate with a mint leaf.

Serve immediately while warm.

Las cosas claras y el chocolate espeso... Ideas should be clear and chocolate thick.

DID YOU KNOW?

Due to its theobromine content, chocolate is toxic to most animals, with the exception of horses. Because it acts as a potent stimulant for horses, its use has been banned in horse-racing.

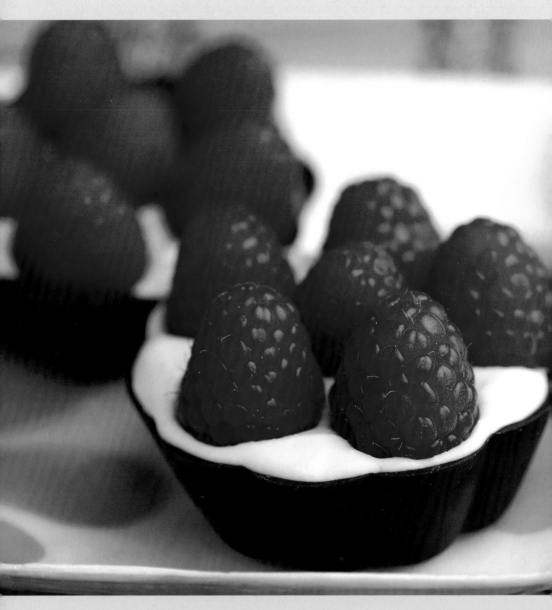

Tester Comments

"Raspberries, cream and chocolate…a heavenly combination, and such a fast impressive dessert to serve my guests."

GF WF NF

RASPBERRY CRÈME CUPS

These elegant cups are a quick,easy, creamy delight...for a treat anytime fresh berries are available!

Makes: 4 - 8 servings (1-2 per person)

8	**dark, dairy-free chocolate cups** (commercially purchased)
2 cups (500 ml)	**SILKY CREAMY WHIPPED TOPPING - Section 3**
40	**large fresh raspberries**

Fill cups with Silky Creamy Whipped Topping (either by spooning or piping).

Decorate with fresh raspberries. Serve immediately, or prepare in advance and refrigerate until serving time.

VARIATION

▶ Replace berries with blackberries or other types.

Chocolate brings to mind marvelous
gratification:
Children......relish it
Lovers......share it
Chocoholics......stash it
Stockbrokers......dabble in it
Wealthy people......lavish in it
Pregnant women......crave it
Designers......market it
Women......need it
Sensualists......indulge in it
Pagans......worship it
Hedonists......enjoy it
Everyone......eats it
~Elaine Sherman
"Chocolate: The Exquisite Indulgence"© 1995 by Running Press

Chocolate has long been considered an aphrodisiac, however there is no conclusive scientific evidence. Interestingly, according to a 2006 Redbook survey, 70% of women prefer chocolate over sex. (Globe & Mail, Feb.10th 2007)

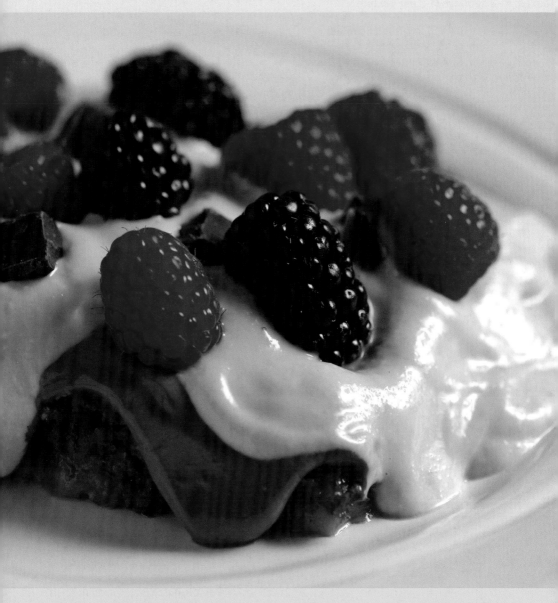

Tester Comments

"Wow…this is tooooo good to be true!"
"Ooooww yeah!"
"Everything to be loved in this decadent, divine, orgasmic, experience."

PASSION IN A PAN

Yes…this is the healthy version of another popular recipe…and there's nothing less decadent about it. Enjoy the "out of this world" experience, while benefiting from a lot less calories!

Makes: One 9"x 14" cake

Fruit bottom:

3-4 cups (750-1000 ml)	**fresh peaches or strawberries, sliced** (or 2-14 oz cans peaches or pineapple tidbits - reserve juice)

Cake Batter:

1 cup (250 ml)	**whole grain pastry flour**
½ cup (125 ml)	**raw sugar** (eg. Sucanat™)
½ tsp (2 ml)	**baking powder**
½ tsp (2 ml)	**baking soda**
½ tsp (2 ml)	**salt**
⅓ cup (75 ml)	**olive oil or melted coconut oil**
1 tsp (5 ml)	**pure vanilla**
¾ cup (150 ml)	**fruit juice** (or reserved juice from canned fruit)
1 cup (250 ml)	**pecans, chopped**

Pudding:
One of the following pudding recipes - Section 2:
▶ **RICH CHOCOLATE MOUSSE**
▶ **INSTANT CHOCOLATE PUDDING**
▶ **QUICK CREAMY AVOCADO CUSTARD**

Preheat oven to 375°F. Grease the bottom and sides of a 9" x 14" pan. Pour the fruit evenly over the bottom of the pan.

In a large bowl, measure the dry ingredients and stir together. Make a well in the middle and add wet ingredients into the center. Mix until all dry ingredients are moist. Fold in chopped nuts.

Spread the batter evenly over the fruit. Bake for 18-20 minutes until golden brown on top. Cool completely.

Make one of the pudding recipes from Section 2 choices.

Note: RICH CHOCOLATE MOUSSE should be made in advance and allowed to cool completely before spreading on cake, whereas the other two can be made and immediately spread over cooled cake. All are delicious, however Chocolate Mousse is the "richest" (and most decadent) of the three choices.

Spread a thick layer of pudding over cooled cake and decorate, if desired with a layer of dried coconut, fresh strawberries or raspberries, more peaches or any other fruit of your choice, or chopped pieces of a chocolate bar.

VARIATION

▶ For an even more decadent dessert, you can also add a layer of SILKY WHIPPED CREAMY TOPPING - Section 2 or commercially purchased Whipped Soy Topping

Chocolate flows in deep dark, sweet waves, a river to ignite my mind and alert my senses.

"According to researchers at the University of Texas Southwestern Medical Center in Dallas, the same antioxidant properties found in red wine that protect against heart disease and possibly cancer are also found in chocolate."

from **Health by Chocolate** *foreword*
by John Robbins

SECTION #3
FILLINGS, FROSTINGS, GLAZES & SYRUP

FRUIT GLAZE/SAUCE [GF WF NF SF RWV]

2 cups (500 ml)	**fresh or frozen juicy fruit** (i.e. peaches, mango, etc)
2-4 Tbsp (30-60 ml)	**pure maple syrup**
1 tsp (5ml)	**pure vanilla**
1 tsp-1 Tbsp (5ml-15 ml)	**kuzu or arrowroot powder**

Blend together fruit, syrup and vanilla in a blender to desired texture. To use as glaze, spoon it on the cake as soon as it comes out of the oven so it can "set". If you want a thickened "jelly-like" fruit sauce, for every 2 cups of juicy fruit, add 1 tsp - 1 Tbsp of thickener and simmer over medium heat until dissolved. Cool to thicken.

Note: Alternately, use a can of unsweetened fruit (eg. mandarin oranges, pears, peaches) and add berries or other chopped fresh fruit.

SIMPLE CHOCOLATE SYRUP [GF WF NF SF]

Use this easy syrup for Chocolate Milk, Ice Cream Topping, Knickerbocker Glory Parfait, Pineapple-Banana Pecan Divinity, or anywhere you need a drizzle of chocolate.

Makes: 12 ounces

1 cup (250 ml)	**water**
1 Tbsp (15 ml)	**arrowroot** (or kuzu)
½ cup (125 ml)	**pure honey**
¼ cup (60 ml)	**cocoa powder**

In a medium saucepan dissolve arrowroot powder in water. Add honey and cocoa and whisk over medium-high heat until thickened (approximately 3-5 minutes).
Use warm over ice cream or cool and refrigerate.

Once completely cooled you can store it in a squeeze bottle for easy drizzlin' (I use a plastic honey container).

Note: Keeps well in refrigerator.

VARIATION
▶ Replace honey with pure maple syrup or agave nectar.

CASHEW COCONUT CREAM `GF WF SF RW`

Use as a frosting or a filling for cakes or crepes, or as a rich delicious soy-free whipped creamy topping on fruit salad.

Makes: Approximately 2 cups

1 cup (250 ml)	**cashews**
⅓ cup (75 ml)	**moist dates**
1-2 tsp (10 ml)	**pure vanilla extract**
½ cup (125 ml)	**coconut milk**
2 Tbsp (30 ml)	**cocoa powder** (optional)

Note: If dates have become too dry, soak them for several minutes in hot water and drain.

Place cashews, dates, vanilla and cocoa powder in a food processor and blend for several minutes. Pour the coconut milk into processor slowly and continue to process for several minutes until you have a thick creamy texture.

Refrigerate for 15 minutes to allow mixture to thicken enough to use as a cake frosting on a cooled cake.

VARIATION

▸ Omit coconut milk and replace dates with ½ cup (125 ml) maple syrup.

▸ Replace nuts with ¾ cups (175 ml) nut butter or tahini.

CHOCOLATE CRÈME FROSTING `GF WF NF`

12 oz (349g)	**silken tofu** (soft or firm)
1½ cups (395 ml)	**melted chocolate chips**

Blend or whip together tofu and melted chocolate. Add variation if desired and cool. Frost a cooled cake by spreading evenly, and decorate.

VARIATION

▸ ZESTY ORANGE: add ¼ cup (60 ml) of orange juice concentrate and 2 Tbsp (30 ml) grated orange zest and ½ tsp (2 ml) cinnamon (optional).

▸ ESPRESSO: add 2 Tbsp (30 ml) cooled espresso <u>or</u> 1 tsp (5 ml) instant coffee granules dissolved in 2 Tbsp (30 ml) hot water to the Chocolate Crème Frosting.

▸ MINT: add 4 finely minced fresh mint leaves, <u>or</u> 2 tsp (10 ml) mint extract to frosting.

CARAMEL FROSTING `GF WF SF RW`

⅓ cup (75 ml)	**macadamia cashew butter**
⅓ cup (75 ml)	**maple syrup, honey or brown rice syrup**

Whip together nut butter and sweetener in a food processor for <u>several minutes</u> until thick like caramel.

SILKY WHIPPED CREAMY TOPPING   GF WF

This is a great topping for pancakes, crepes, cakes, pudding, custards, pies, ice cream and parfaits.

Makes: Approximately 2 cups

½ cup (125 ml)	**maple syrup**
½ cup (125 ml)	**cashews**
1 tsp (5 ml)	**lemon juice**
12 oz (349 g)	**medium-firm silken tofu**
1 Tbsp (15 ml)	**pure vanilla**

Optional:

1 tsp (5 ml) **agar powder** <u>or</u> **2 tsp** (10 ml**) agar flakes** <u>plus</u> **¼ cup** (60 ml) **water**

Note: Agar is a vegetarian jello derived from sea vegetable found in health markets. The agar and water can be omitted, however the agar gives it a lighter "Cool Whip™" texture. If using the optional agar and water, stir together in a small saucepan. Bring to a boil over medium heat and simmer for 4-5 minutes until agar is dissolved. Add maple syrup to saucepan and stir (the syrup will help to cool down the mixture).

In a blender or food processor, blend cashews, lemon juice and tofu until creamy. Add contents of saucepan and vanilla and blend until incorporated, scraping sides of processor if necessary.

Serve immediately or store in refrigerator. Will keep for at least 7 days.

VARIATION

▸ For a quicker version omit agar and water and simply add the maple syrup to the remaining ingredients.

▸ Replace vanilla with ½ tsp (2 ml) mint <u>or</u> orange extract or ¾ cup (175 ml) berries and 2 tsp (10 ml) lemon juice <u>or</u> ¼ cup (60 ml) of cocoa powder.

▸ Use your imagination by adding: cinnamon, cardamom or other spices.

Note: Use silken tofu in tetra pak. For the **thickest** creme, use firm silken tofu. For a **thinner** creme, use (soft or medium) silken tofu. If silken is unavailable, soft or medium <u>fresh</u> tofu can be substituted.

TOFU MAPLE CAKE ICING   GF WF

A dependable stand-by, always popular on cakes, cupcakes and other delights.

Makes: 2½ cups

8 oz (250 g)	**tofu, firm silken**
1 cup (250 ml)	**cashew butter**
¾-1 cup	**pure maple syrup**
2 tsp (10 ml)	**vanilla**

Blend all ingredients in a food processor, using the 'S' blade.

Note: The variation of syrup amount depends on the oiliness of the cashew butter. Aim for a thicker frosting that will spread easily.

"People with heart problems are sometimes told to take a baby aspirin a day. The reason is that aspirin thins the blood and reduces the likelihood of clots forming (clots play a key role in many heart attacks and strokes). Research…found that chocolate also thins the blood, and performs the same anti-clotting activity as aspirin."

*from **Health by Chocolate** foreword*
by John Robbins

SECTION #4
CAKES & COOKIES, BARS & BONBONS

Sweet-More Bars
pg. 77

Dark Chocolate
Macaroons
pg. 79

Cocoa Millet Chews
pg. 81

Macadamia Nut
Truffles
pg. 83

No-Bake Chocolate
Drops
pg. 85

Crunchy Munchie
Chocolate Chip Cookies
pg. 87

Raspberry Chocolate
Oat Bars
pg. 89

Healthy
Turtle Bonbons
pg. 91

Triple Omega
Energy Balls
pg. 93

Sesame Ginger
Black Ball Bliss
pg. 95

Almond Coconut
Joy Bars
pg. 97

Chocolate
Cheezecake
pg. 99

Chocolate Ginger
Pecan Pie
pg. 101

Double Double Chocolate
Fudge Brownies
pg. 103

Black Forest
Cherry Torte
pg. 105

Cranberry Nut
Chocolate Chip Muffins
pg. 107

Spicy Chocolate
Gingerbread Cake
pg. 109

Orange Chocolate Cake
with Zesty Crème Frosting
pg. 111

Celebration Mandala
pg. 113

DID YOU KNOW?

Peanuts aren't actually in the nut family but are legumes along with kidney and pinto beans. Peanuts are a good source of protein.

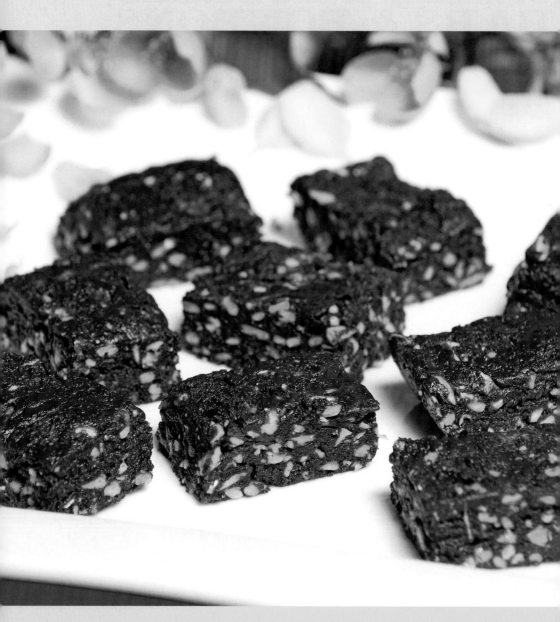

Tester Comments

"Ten out of ten. Makes me want to eat more."
"We love the peanut butter chocolate combo."
"The kids love this."

SWEET-MORE BARS

These taste similar to EAT-MORE® bars. They are very fast to make with minimal mess; one pot and one measuring cup…that's it! Kids of any age love these tried-and-true treats.

Makes: 20 bars

1 cup (250 ml)	**peanut butter**
1 cup (250 ml)	**honey** (or brown rice syrup)
1 cup (250 ml)	**cocoa or carob powder** (or ½ cup of each)
1 cup (250 ml)	**unsweetened shredded coconut**
1 cup (250 ml)	**sunflower or sesame seeds** (or ½ cup of each)
1 Tbsp (15 ml)	**coconut butter** (to grease pan)

In a heavy saucepan, heat honey and peanut butter until bubbly. Add cocoa powder, seeds and coconut.

Grease a 9" x 9" pan, and press mixture firmly into pan.

Cool completely and cut into bars or squares.

VARIATION

► Can be cooled slightly and rolled into balls instead of squares bars.

All I really need is love, but a little chocolate now
and then doesn't hurt! ~ Lucy Van Pelt
(Peanuts - by Charles M. Schulz)

DID YOU KNOW?

The processing of Dutch cocoa powder, due to the alkali used to neutralized its natural acidity, reduces the amount of healthful flavanoids.

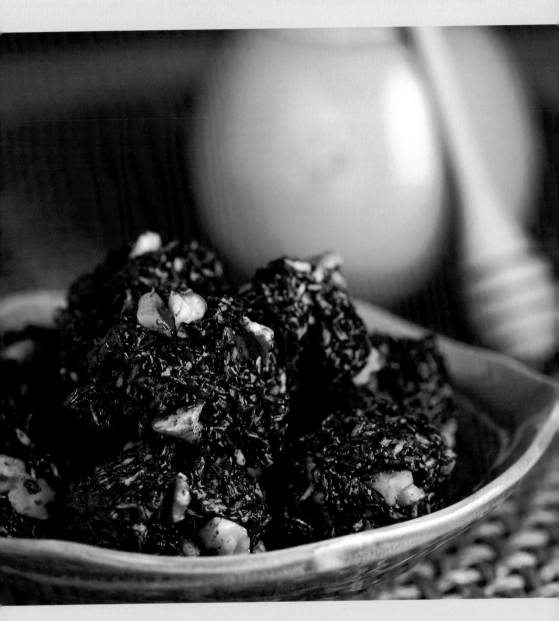

Tester Comments

"Wow, egg-free and more delicious!"
"I loved the sweet-nutty, chewy combination…mmm!"

DARK CHOCOLATE MACAROONS

I developed this egg-free version that always satisfies a sweet tooth and chocolate craving. They make a good treat for traveling.

Makes: approximately 3 dozen

¾ cup (175 ml)	**honey**
¾ cup (175 ml)	**dark cocoa powder**
2 cups (500 ml)	**dried, unsweetened coconut**
¾ cup (175 ml)	**coarsely chopped walnuts**

VARIATION

▸ Replace walnuts with sunflower seeds.

▸ Form macaroons into "birds' nests" by molding an indent with your wet thumb or the back of a spoon. Fill each nest with jellybean "eggs" or other treats.

Prepare a cookie sheet or tray with a layer of waxed paper or grease with coconut oil.

Chop and measure nuts.

Measure cocoa powder and honey into a heavy saucepan.

Helpful Hint: When measuring honey, lightly oil the measuring cup so honey pours out more easily.

Mix well and stir over medium-low heat until bubbly and simmer approx. 2-3 minutes.

Remove from heat and add coconut and nuts. Cool several minutes (enough for handling).

Drop by teaspoons onto the prepared cookie sheet and let sit for at least half an hour to set.

I could give up chocolate, but I'm not a quitter.

DID YOU KNOW?

Millet is a high protein grain, eaten by healthy people and canaries.

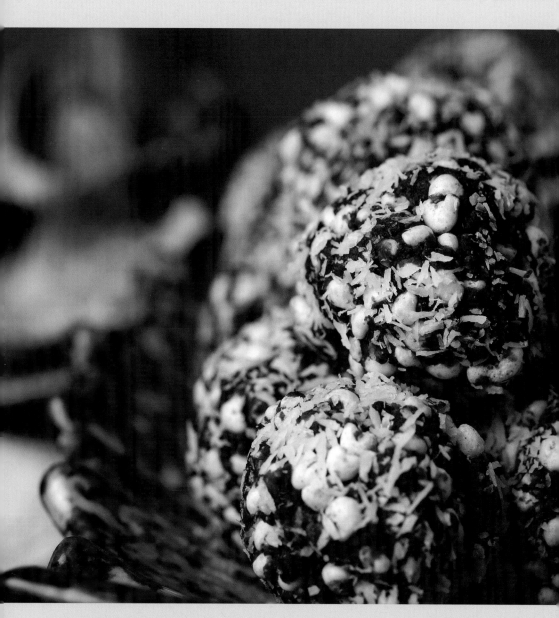

Tester Comments

"This recipe was easy to follow and prepare as cookies or squares and the kids liked them as a replacement for Rice Crispy squares."

"Quick and easy preparation."

"Putting them in a pan is much faster than rolling them into balls, although rolling them into balls doesn't take that long."

COCOA-MILLET CHEWS

These are a hit with everyone! In fact they're a best seller at Edmonton's Organic Roots Food Market where I first developed the recipe. The pure carob version has an incredibly delicious "chocolatey" taste if you want a non-chocolate chew. Healthy enough to be a "snack"...decadent enough to be a "treat".

Makes: approx. 18-24 balls or squares

1 cup (250 ml)	**almond, cashew or other nut butter**
½ **cup** (125 ml)	**honey, pure maple syrup or brown rice syrup**
1 tsp (5 ml)	**pure vanilla extract**
¼ **cup** (60 ml)	**chocolate or carob powder** (or some of each)
2½ -3 cups (625 - 750 ml)	**puffed millet cereal** (or other wholegrain puffed cereal)
¾ **cup** (175 ml)	**dried unsweetened coconut**

Optional additions:

½ **cup** (125 ml)	**chopped nuts or seeds**
½ **cup** (125 ml)	**chocolate or carob chips**
½ **cup** (125 ml)	**dried fruit** (eg. raisins, cranberries, chopped apricots, dates)
½ **tsp** (2 ml)	**ground cinnamon or ground cardamom**

Heat nut butter and sweetener over medium heat for approximately 2-3 minutes, stirring constantly until mixture is just beginning to bubble.

Take off heat and stir in vanilla.

Mix in cocoa or carob powder, cereal and any of the other optional additions. Incorporate coconut if making bars, or set aside for rolling into balls.

Cool several minutes until safe enough to handle.

Squares or Bars:
Press into 8" x 10" greased or lined pan. Cool and cut into squares before serving.

Balls:
Mold into balls (approximately ½ cup (125 ml) or more) and roll in coconut. Cool on counter or in refrigerator until firm (approximately 10 minutes).

Life without chocolate is like
a beach without water.

Macadamia nuts are high in fat, mostly unsaturated. They are good sources of magnesium and potassium, and contain thiamine, zinc, iron, copper, niacin and phosphorus.

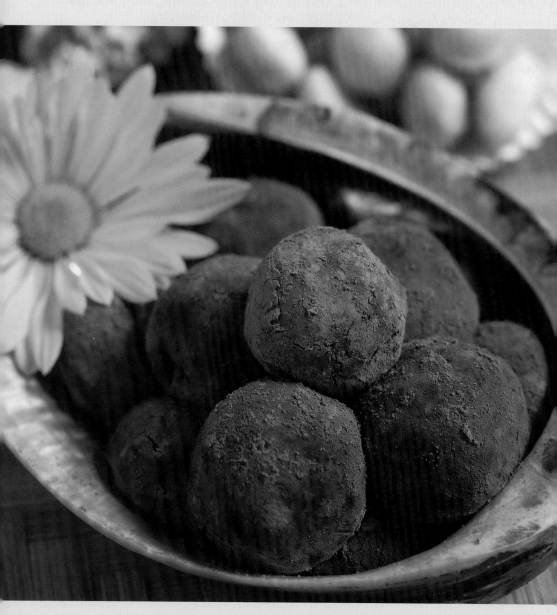

Tester Comments

"Much better than those chocolate covered macadamia nuts you get in Hawaii."
"Oh wow… these are scrumptious!"

MACADAMIA NUT TRUFFLES

Oooo lala...these are marvelous morsels that make wonderful gifts...make a batch for yourself and a batch to give away. They can also be frozen.

Makes: 20-26 truffles

½ **cup** (125 ml)	**pure maple syrup**
½ **cup** (125 ml)	**macadamia nuts**
½ **cup** (125 ml)	**almond flour meal** (finely ground blanched almonds)
¼ **cup** (60 ml)	**cocoa powder**
2 Tbsp (30 ml)	**coconut milk**
¼ **cup** (60 ml)	**cocoa powder to roll truffles**

Note: You can purchase almond flour/meal at health food markets or make your own by grinding blanched almonds.

VARIATION
- ▶ Replace macadamia nuts with cashews.
- ▶ Replace almonds with hazelnuts.

Put the maple syrup in a heavy pot and bring to a boil.

In a food processor with the 'S' blade, pulse the macadamia nuts until they are finely ground.

When syrup has boiled for approximately 3-5 minutes, add the almond flour meal and ground nuts. Continue to allow the syrup to thicken, stirring frequently, until mixture is almost dry and nuts are all sticking together (syrup is not runny). Add the cocoa powder and coconut milk, stirring well. Remove from heat.

Scrape truffle mixture into a container and place in the fridge to cool.

When mixture has cooled (approximately 20-30 minutes), roll into ping-pong size balls or smaller, and roll each ball in dry cocoa powder to coat.

Store in an airtight container in the fridge. These will keep for several weeks if you hide them well.

Nobody knows the truffles I've seen!

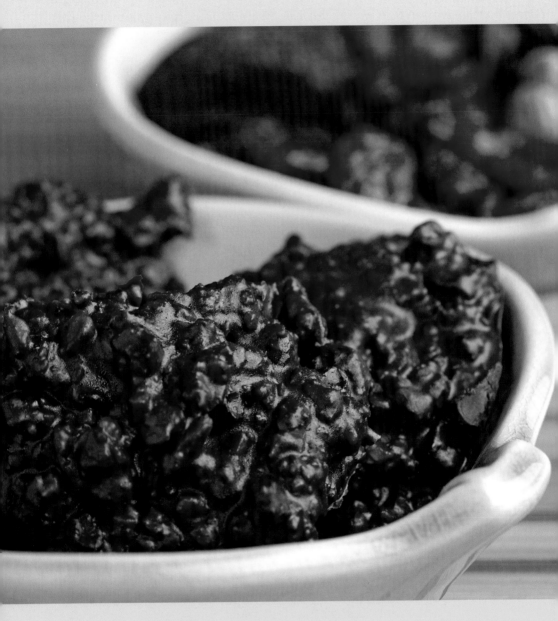

Tester Comments

"I love experimenting with different fruits, nuts and spices...a new combination every time."

NO BAKE CHOCOLATE DROPS

If you can't find the chocolate bar flavour you're craving here's an easy solution! Use a high cocoa, low sugar content bar, drops or chips to melt with your favourite flavour. One of my favourites - toasted almonds and freshly ground anise.

Makes: Amount varies depending on ingredients used

1 cup (250 ml)   **dark chocolate chips**
(or 100 gm dark melting chocolate - I use 72% Cooks Chocolate)

YOUR CHOICE OF:
(amount will vary)

Dried Fruit: **raisins, figs, prunes, blueberries, apricots, cranberries, goji berries, etc.**

Nuts Seeds: **pecans, walnuts, dry roasted almonds, macadamia, sunflower seeds, pumpkin seeds, etc.**

Spices: **ground cinnamon, ground cardamom, ground star anise, grated ginger root or ginger powder, chili powder, lemon zest, etc.**

Be adventurous: you may be pleasantly surprised!

Note: To dry roast nuts, spread them onto a baking sheet and place in a preheated 400°F oven for 4-7 minutes until lightly toasted. Check often as they can burn quickly!

Line a baking sheet, or flat tray or plate with waxed or parchment paper.

Chop nuts and fruit into medium or small pieces. Melt chocolate - See rules in section ABOUT RECIPES. Remove from heat and add the desired additions.

Drop into mounds or spread flat. Press with the back of a metal spoon or with moistened hands to desired thickness.

Cool and break or cut into wedges of desired size.

Store in a ziplock bag or container in your secret hiding place.

Note: Freezing is the fastest way to "set" this creation...(and who wants to wait!).

The first chocolate bar mould was invented in 1847.

Whole grains and whole grain flour contain the beneficial "germ" and "bran" layers, which are no longer present in refined white flour. The germ is high in healthful fatty acids and the bran contains beneficial dietary fibre. Whole grains also provide far more flavour than refined.

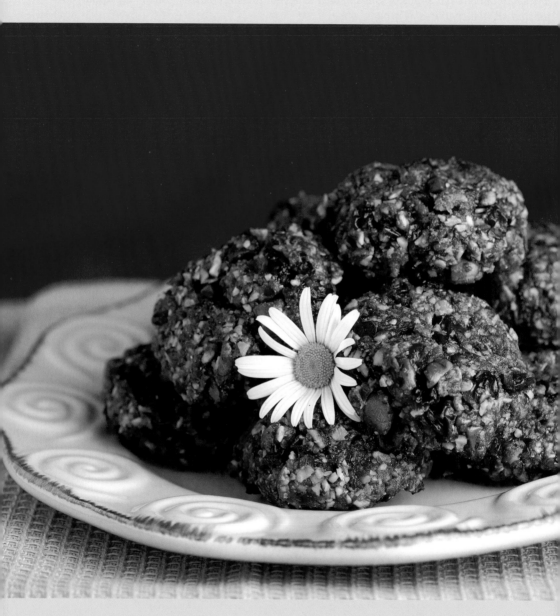

Tester Comments

"These were fantastic. My husband even managed to convince me they constitute quality "breakfast food" and I had no way to argue, given the ingredients."

"I don't much care for dates so I didn't want to try them. But I was surprised at how good these really are."

"These are the cat's meow!"

GFV WFV SF

CRUNCHY MUNCHIE CHOCOLATE CHIP COOKIES OR BARS

These delicious, sturdy cookies pack well in lunches or for trips.

Makes: 2 dozen cookies

1¼ cups (300 ml)	**dates, pitted**
2 tsp (10 ml)	**vanilla**
½ cup (125 ml)	**nut butter**
¾ cup (175 ml)	**rolled oats**
¾ cup (175 ml)	**whole grain flour**
1½ cups (375 ml)	**dried fruit** (eg. raisins, cranberries, cherries, blueberries, chopped apricots)
½ cup (125 ml)	**sunflower seeds**
½ cup (125 ml)	**chopped pecans**
1 cup (250 ml)	**chocolate or carob chips** (or ½ cup of nibs)

Flax Gel:

3 Tbsp (45 ml)	**flax seeds** (whole or previously ground)
½ cup (125 ml)	**water**

VARIATION

▶ Change up the fruit and nuts or seeds as desired.

▶ Use brown rice flour and gluten free flakes for a gluten free version.

Preheat oven to 325°F.

Grind dates and vanilla in a food processor or with a wooden spoon. Cream in the nut butter.

Mix in remaining ingredients, except the flax gel.

Make flax gel and fold into cookie mixture.

FLAX GEL: Grind 3 Tbsp whole flax seeds in coffee spice grinder. With a blender or hand blender, whip together ground seeds with ½ cup of water until an egg white consistency is achieved.

Drop by spoonfuls close together on greased baking sheets or a greased 9"x13" baking pan.

Bake for 10-12 minutes for cookies, or until peaks begin to brown. Bake 25-30 minutes for bars. Cool and serve.

*Some say women are addicted to chocolate...
I say we're merely loyal.*

Raspberries are high in dietary fibre, vitamin C and bioflavanoids. They can help relieve heartburn and constipation.

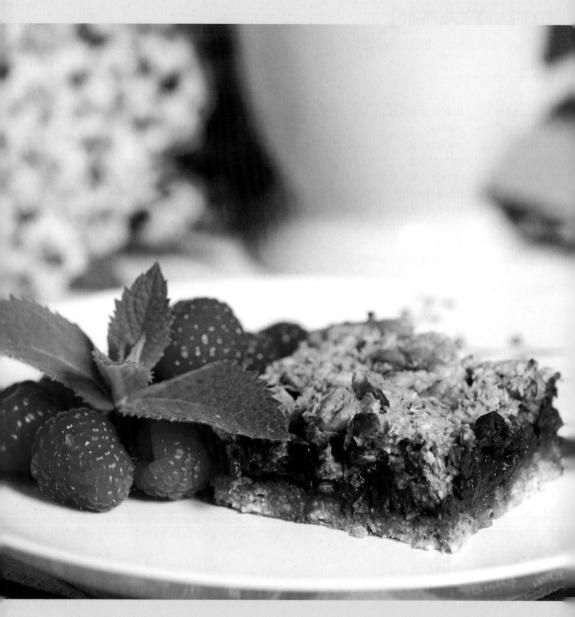

Tester Comments

"These got five 10/10's in my office."

RASPBERRY CHOCOLATE OAT BARS

Can't get your kids to eat their oatmeal? They won't skip breakfast with these in the house. Quick and yummy with a sweet surprise center!

Makes: 12 bars

1-1¼ cups (250-300 ml)	**large ripe bananas** (2-3)	Preheat oven to 350°F.
2 cups (500 ml)	**oat flakes or quick oats**	Mash bananas. Mix together all ingredients except jam and chocolate chips. Flatten half the batter into a 9" x 9" greased baking pan.
1 tsp (5 ml)	**salt**	
½-1 tsp (5 ml)	**coriander or cinnamon**	Spread with raspberry jam, sprinkle with chocolate chips, and spoon remaining batter over top, spreading with the back of a large metal spoon.
pinch	**cloves** (optional)	
½ cup (125 ml)	**chopped walnuts**	
1 cup (250 ml)	**unsweetened dry coconut**	Bake for 25-30 minutes until lightly browned.
⅓ cup (75 ml)	**pure maple syrup or pure honey or agave nectar**	Serve warm or cooled.
¾-1 cup (175-250 ml)	**raspberry jam**	Slice into squares or bars.
¾-1 cup (175-250 ml)	**dark chocolate chips**	Keep leftovers in fridge.

VARIATION

▶ Replace raspberry jam with mashed berries sweetened with 2 Tbsp (30 ml) pure maple syrup or honey.

▶ Oat flakes are chewier and have higher fibre content.

▶ Replace walnuts with pecans, sunflower seeds or slivered almonds.

Love chocolate completely, without complexes or false shame; remember, "there is no reasonable man without a spark of madness."

~ François de La Rochefoucauld (1630-1680)

DID YOU KNOW?

Dates are high in potassium, and are a source of pantothenic acid, vitamin B6, and niacin, iron, magnesium and other minerals. There are many varieties of dates. They should be purchased plump, soft and well colored. Dull looking fruit can be too dried out.

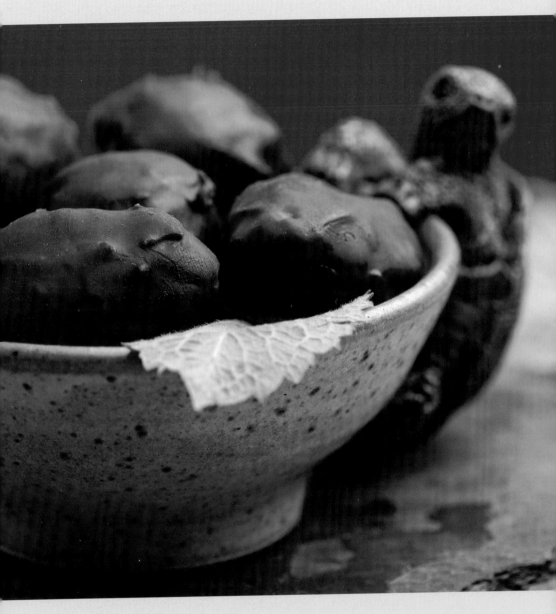

Tester Comments

"Just sweet enough for my afternoon tea!"
"Finger lickin' good."

HEALTHY TURTLE BONBONS

Like the famous chocolate candy, these chewy treats are sweet and decadent with a surprising, pleasing crunch, and so easy to make.

Makes: 12 turtle bonbons

12	**whole medjool dates**
	(or other large dates)
12	**whole pecans or walnuts**
¾ **cup** (175 ml)	**dark chocolate chips**

Line a tray or flat plate with waxed or parchment paper or plastic wrap.

With your fingers, remove pit from each date, and replace it with a nut. Gently squeeze the date closed around the nut.

Melt chocolate - See rules in section ABOUT RECIPES.

Roll each stuffed date in chocolate using a fork or tongs.

Place individual treats on the prepared tray so they don't touch, and allow to cool and set on the counter or, if the room is warm, in the fridge.

When coating has hardened, serve on a glass or decorative plate or in individual small baking cups or candy holders.

VARIATION

▶ For those who love the bitterness of cocoa powder and want an extra edge, roll each chocolate coated turtle in cocoa powder. (**Note**: they lose their glossy look).

— *Toasted almonds*

Money talks, chocolate sings.

Flax seeds, hemp seeds and walnuts are of the highest plant sources of omega-3 fatty acids. The lignans in flax can help to reduce or eliminate hot flashes in menopausal women. Grinding the flax seeds breaks down the shell more easily than chewing, and allows more healthy fat to be available.

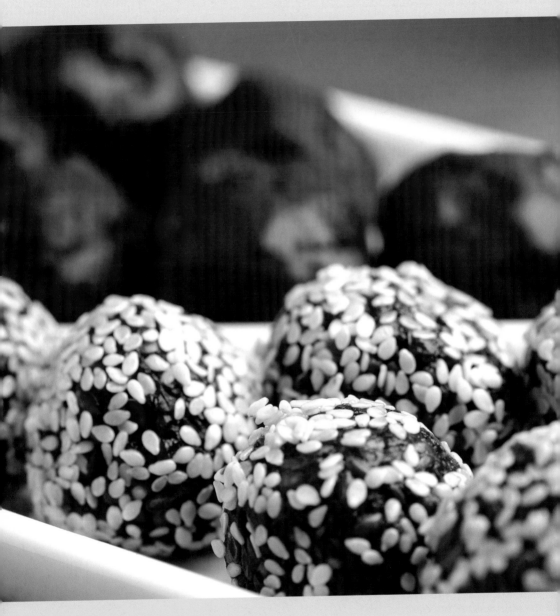

Tester Comments

"I like the light nutty taste. Perfect finger food."
"These do keep you going…lots of energy after a few of these tasty morsels…and inexpensive compared to 'nutrition' bars."

TRIPLE OMEGA ENERGY BALLS

Preparing for a long afternoon or day ahead? These will provide energy for the long haul, and make a yummy breakfast or snack on the run.

Makes: 16 ping-pong sized balls

2 Tbsp (30 ml)	**flax seeds** (ground or unground)
2 Tbsp (30 ml)	**hulled hemp seeds**
1 cup (250 ml)	**walnuts**
¾ cup (175 ml)	**apricots**
¾ cup (175 ml)	**figs or raisins**
¼ cup (60 ml)	**cocoa powder**
2 Tbsp (30 ml)	**cocoa nibs** (optional)
½ -1 tsp (5 ml)	**maca, ginseng or cinnamon**
¼ cup (60 ml)	**white sesame seeds** (or hulled hemp seeds or ground coconut flakes)
½ cup (125 ml)	**chocolate chips for melting** (optional)

Note: You need moist dried fruits for this recipe. If they are too dried out, soak them in hot water for several minutes to soften and re-hydrate. Drain water before using.

If grinding flax seeds, place in a spice coffee grinder and pulse several times.

Place all ingredients, except sesame seeds and chocolate chips into a food processor and process several minutes (usually at least two) with an 'S' blade, until mixture forms a moist mass.

Roll mixture into balls and set on a plate.

Quickly dip each ball in a bowl of water and roll in the sesame seeds to coat or in melted chocolate - See rules in section ABOUT RECIPES.

Refrigerate any leftovers.

VARIATION

▶ Add other health building ingredients, for example, goji berries, spirulina, greens powder, etc. instead of, or as well as, maca or ginseng.

Simply put...everyone has a price, mine is chocolate!

DID YOU KNOW?

Black sesame seeds are very flavourful, and while usually more expensive, are well worth it. Sesame seeds are high in calcium, magnesium, potassium, iron, zinc, thiamine, niacin, folic acid, vitamin B6, and are a great source of dietary fibre. They are beneficial for the nervous system, used to aid digestion and help to activate blood circulation. The nutrients in sesame seeds are better assimilated by the body when consumed as paste butter called tahini.

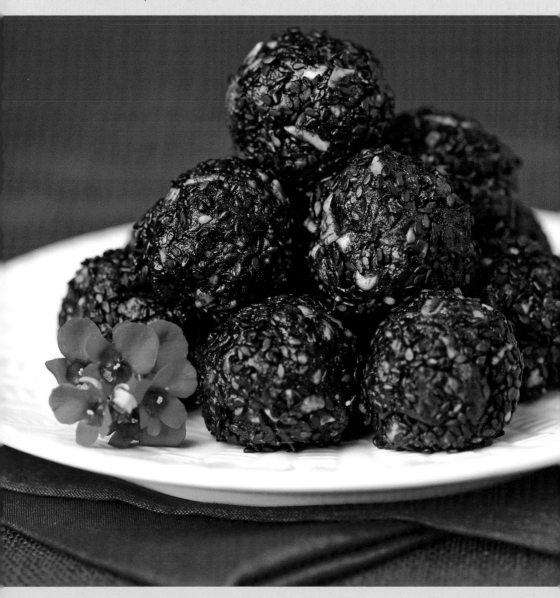

Tester Comments

"I especially enjoyed the harmonious blend of an entire orchard of natural ingredients."
"Consistency of the raw batter made it easy to make the balls."

SESAME GINGER "BLACK BALL BLISS"

I think ginger and sesame have an affinity for each other. I invented these for a Baha'i celebration where our friend Jean kept referring to "those delicious little black balls".

Makes: 16-20 balls

6	**dried apricots, finely chopped**
⅓ **cup** (75 ml)	**dried candied ginger, finely chopped**
1 cup (250 ml)	**sunflower seeds, ground**
½ **cup** (125 ml)	**tahini** (sesame seed butter)
¼ **cup** (60 ml)	**cocoa powder**
4	**large pitted dates**
¼ **cup** (60 ml)	**cocoa nibs** (optional)
⅓ **cup** (75 ml)	**black sesame seeds** (or, if unavailable white sesame seeds)

Chop apricots and ginger and set aside.

In a food processor, grind together the seeds, tahini, cocoa powder and dates until smooth.

Transfer to a bowl and add dried apricots and ginger (and optional cocoa nibs) and fold together. Shape into balls and roll in black sesame seeds.

VARIATION

▶ Can also be made into a large ball, and used as a paté for crackers.

"To eat chocolate, or not to eat chocolate...there is NO question".

~ Geri "Shakespeare" Norris

Brazil nuts are very high in selenium, an antioxidant nutrient that helps prevent cancers and aging. Joy is helpful in preventing cancer too!

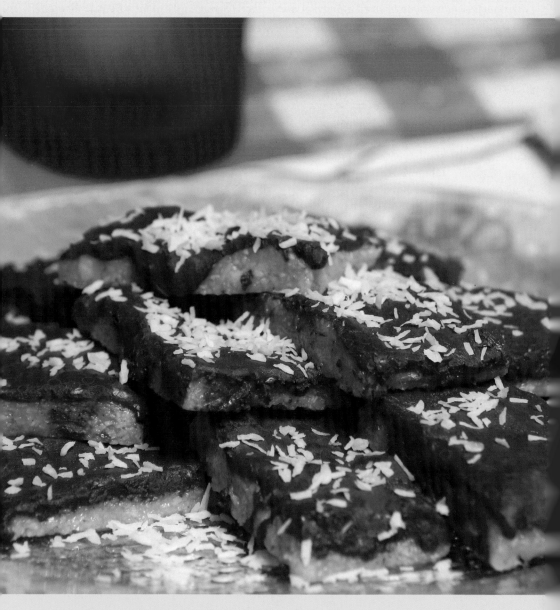

Tester Comments

"These were so good that my husband didn't get to try them because I ate all the samples Victoria gave me to take home!"

"Quick and easy to make, and storage isn't an issue with these…they get eaten too fast!"

ALMOND COCONUT JOY BARS

Oh Joy!! These bars are sweet and decadent and a big hit with everyone I've served them to. ENJOY!

Makes: 25 - 35 depending on size

½ - ¾ **cup** (125-175 ml)	**Brazil nuts, coarsely chopped**
1 cup (250 ml)	**pure honey** (or brown rice syrup)
1½ **cups** (375 ml)	**dried unsweetened coconut**
1½ **cups** (375 ml)	**almond flour meal**
¾ **cup** (175 ml)	**chocolate chips**

VARIATION

▸ Replace Brazil nuts with chopped almonds.

Note: Almond "flour meal" can be purchased commercially in health food markets or made in a food processor with blanched almonds using the 'S' blade.

Line a cookie sheet with waxed or parchment paper. Coarsely chop the Brazil nuts by hand or in the food processor, pulsing a few times.

In a large saucepan heat honey over medium heat. Reduce heat to simmer for approx. 3-4 minutes, until thickened. Add the coconut, almond flour meal and chopped nuts.

Remove from heat and spread onto a 9" x 11" lined baking sheet - approximately ½" thick. Smooth out batter with wet fingers. Sprinkle immediately with chocolate chips, allowing them to begin to melt on the warm mixture.

After several minutes smooth the melted chocolate with the back of a spoon or spatula to spread out. Allow to cool in fridge, and cut into small squares or bars.

Does the notion of chocolate preclude
the concept of free will?

~Sandra Boynton

DID YOU KNOW?

Tofu is a high protein food. This combination of whole food ingredients is nutritious enough to use for a meal, along with other balanced meals. Yes, I really do recommend this cheezecake for breakfast! How's that for radical?!

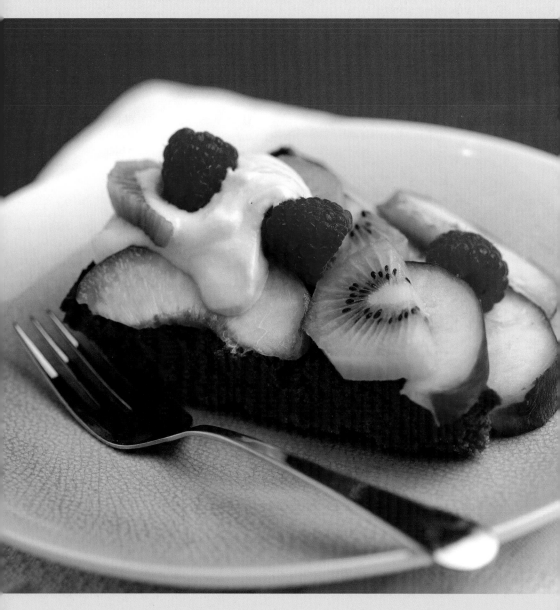

Tester Comments

"A self-proclaimed carnivore in my office said, 'Given what you told me this is made of, I can't believe it tastes this good!'"
"Wow, cheesecake for breakfast!"

CHOCOLATE CHEEZECAKE

There are 349 calories in 100 grams of cream cheese and 62 calories in the same amount of silken firm tofu. Even with the addition of a small amount of almond butter, the fat difference is significant. Cream cheese is 10 times higher in fat with the same protein count. You can replace this nutty crust with a wholegrain flour crust if you prefer. This cheezecake is dense and can be eaten as is, however a fruit topping lightens it up and allows you to vary it each time you make it. They'll never know it's tofu!

Makes: 8 - 12 Servings

Crust:

1 cup (250 ml)	**pecans**
3-4	**large dates, pitted**
⅔ cup (150 ml)	**whole grain flour** (kumut, whole wheat, brown rice, etc.)
⅓ cup (75 ml)	**almond butter**

Filling:

1-15 oz (454 gm)	**pkg medium-firm tofu**
2 Tbsp (30 ml)	**almond butter**
4 large (eg. medjool)	**dates, pitted**
1½ cups (35 ml)	**dark chocolate chips or carob chips, melted**

Your Choice:
▶ **FRUIT GLAZE or SAUCE - Section 3**
▶ **FRESH FRUIT**

CRUST: In a food processor grind pecans and dates together, add in flour and almond butter and pulse until blended. Press firmly into a large cheesecake pan. Preheat oven to 350°F.

FILLING: Melt chocolate - See rules in section ABOUT RECIPES. In a food processor or blender combine filling ingredients, stirring in melted chips. Pour into pan.

Bake for one hour, until filling is firm and doesn't jiggle. If you want your fruit sauce to become a glaze, pour it over the cake as soon as it comes out of the oven; otherwise cool cake completely and add sauce to individual servings.

Optional:
Decorate with a dollop of SILKY WHIPPED CREAMY TOPPING - Section 3

Put the chocolate in the bag and nobody gets hurt.

Raw nuts and dried fruit provide a host of food enzymes, and with ginger as a digestive aid, this healthful "pie-cake" can be enjoyed for celebrations or whenever you want a healthy and decadent treat.

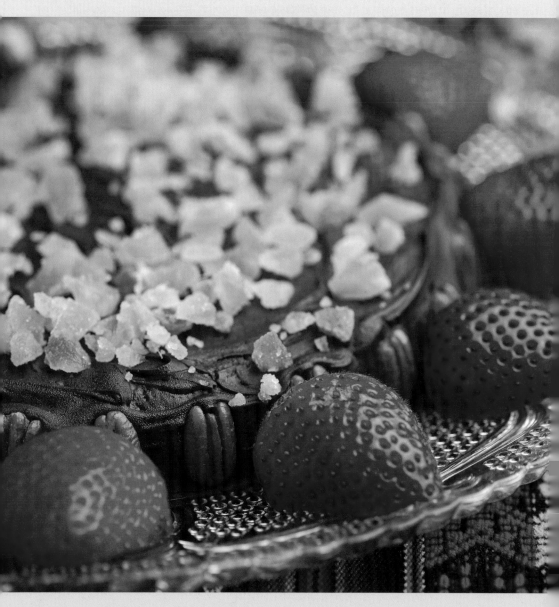

Tester Comments

"This recipe was so simple I read the directions twice to make sure I wasn't missing anything."

"This was really fast and easy...only 10 minutes. It took me longer to find my cheesecake pan then to prepare it."

"Great when company drops over, or you need a special dessert fast."

"This was delicious with tea, not overly sweet."

CHOCOLATE GINGER PECAN PIE

The ginger version of this is my favourite, but it is great with or without. We get the benefit of the natural sweetness, healthy fat and enzymes in the raw nuts and fruit with enough chocolate to satisfy that desire too.

Makes: 12 pieces

2¼ cups (560 ml)	**pecans** (reserve ¼ cup whole pecans for garnish)
2 cups (500 ml)	**pitted dates** (or 1 cup (250 ml) dates and 1 cup (250 ml) raisins)
½ - ¼ cup (125-175 ml)	**chocolate chips or carob chips, melted**
4-6	**large strawberries, sliced** (optional)
1-2 Tbsp (15-30 ml)	**candied ginger, chopped**

In a food processor, grind pecan and date mixture until they form a dough-like mass.

Helpful Hint: Prior to patting the dough mixture into the pan, sprinkle some ground nuts or oat flakes under the pie for easier removal.

Press into a cheesecake pan, pie pan or form with your hands (quickest way) onto a decorative plate.

Melt chocolate - See rules in section ABOUT RECIPES. Mix in the chopped candied ginger or sprinkle over top of pie to decorate. Spread onto pie cake with a knife or the back of a spoon.

Decorate with reserved pecans and fresh strawberries, if desired.

VARIATION

▶ Add ½ cup (125 ml) coconut to dough mixture.

▶ Substitute dates with other dried fruits.

▶ CARAMEL PECAN PIE - To make a crust press the basic pie recipe into the bottom of two small or one large pie pan(s). Fill with a layer of CARAMEL FROSTING - Section 3 and lay the whole pecans on top.

▶ Ginger can be eliminated.

Nine out of ten people like chocolate.
The tenth person always lies...
~John Tullius (1953-)

DID YOU KNOW?

Almonds are a low-fat nut; rich in magnesium and beneficial for muscles, skin, nails, teeth and bones. They are a durable nut that can be stored easily as they are slow to become rancid. Always purchase fresh nuts and seeds.

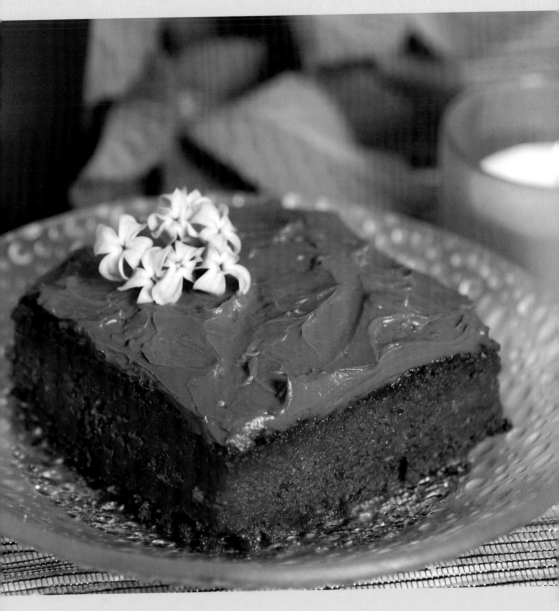

Tester Comments

"Fudgy, moist and delicious...the espresso version is my favourite...or is it the mint?"

"DOUBLE DOUBLE" CHOCOLATE FUDGE BROWNIES

These rich and chewy almond brownies are grain free and "low-glycemic". You can also use this recipe as the base for BLACK FOREST CHERRY TORTE.

Makes: 12-16 brownies

16	**medium-large dates** (or 24 prunes)
¼- ½ cup (60-125 ml)	**water**
1 400 ml (14 oz)	**can coconut milk**
½ cup (125 ml)	**dark cocoa powder**
⅓ cup (75 ml)	**honey**
2 cups (500 ml)	**almond flour**
1 batch	**CHOCOLATE CRÈME FROSTING - Section 3** (Omit for SFV)

Preheat oven to 400ºF.

Simmer dates or prunes in water for 3-5 minutes until moist and plump.

Note: Alternately, use a jar of baby food pureed prunes.

Transfer to a mixing bowl and add coconut milk, cocoa powder and honey. Mix together with a hand blender or transfer to a blender to combine. Mix in almond flour.

Bake in a 9" x 9" greased baking pan for 40-45 minutes.

Cool completely, spread with frosting and cut into squares.

VARIATION

▸ ESPRESSO: See variations for CHOCOLATE CRÈME FROSTING - Section 3.

▸ NUTTY: Sprinkle with ¼ cup (60 ml) chopped nuts (walnuts, pecans or slivered almonds).

▸ MINT: See variations for CHOCOLATE CRÈME FROSTING - Section 3.

The average North American consumes 11.7 pounds of chocolate each year, and the Swiss go through 22.3 pounds yearly.

DID YOU KNOW?

75% of chocolate purchases are made by women, except during the days and minutes prior to Valentine's day, when the tables are turned and 75% of chocolate sales (over $1 billion worth) are made by men!

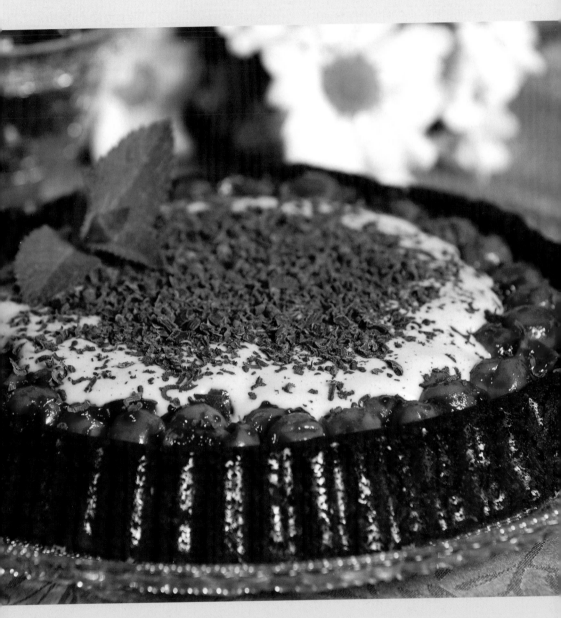

Tester Comments

"I love the fresh, moist combination of cherries and chocolate."
"Such a decadent treat and so very pretty."

BLACK FOREST CHERRY TORTE

DOUBLE DOUBLE CHOCOLATE FUDGE BROWNIE recipe makes the base for this easy torte.

Makes: 6 servings

1 batch	**DOUBLE DOUBLE CHOCOLATE FUDGE BROWNIES** (from previous page)
1½-2 cups (375-500 ml)	**fresh cherries, pitted and chopped or pureed** (or unsweetened canned cherries or cherry jam for a sweeter version)
1 batch	**SILKY WHIPPED CREAMY TOPPING - Section 3**
1 chocolate bar	(optional)

Bake Chocolate Fudge Brownie recipe in a torte pan, or other similar sized baking pan. Allow to cool completely.

Arrange fresh cherries, or spread jam or canned cherries over the torte.

Spread with SILKY WHIPPED CREAMY TOPPING.

Grate chocolate bar using a grater or vegetable peeler. Sprinkle over torte to garnish.

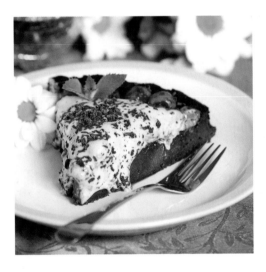

Save the Earth! It's the only planet with chocolate!!

DID YOU KNOW?

High in vitamin C and potassium, the tartness of cranberries is due to their acids. Known for their astringent properties, cranberries and their juice are used in the treatment of urinary tract infections because the berries inhibit bacteria from attaching to the bladder wall.

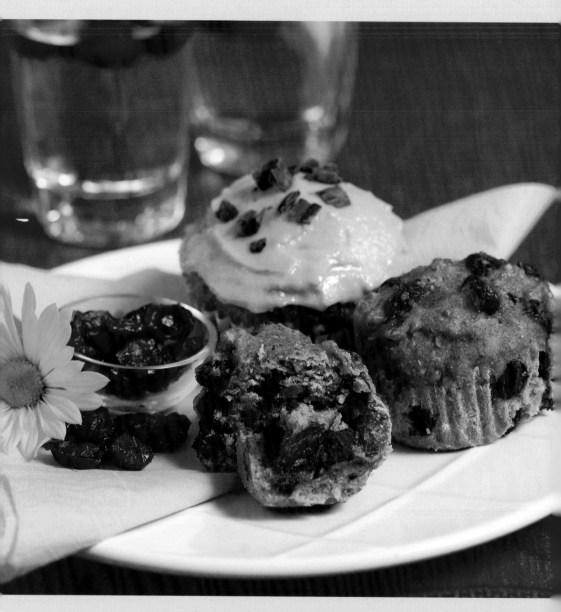

Tester Comments

"I loved these as both cupcakes and muffins."
"The cranberries, chocolate and nuts are a great combination of flavours."

CRANBERRY NUT CHOCOLATE CHIP CUPCAKES

Cranberries, nuts and chocolate…a snazzy combination that is exciting and pleasurable. With or without the frosting, you have a great breakfast muffin.

Makes: 12 cupcakes

1 Tbsp (15 ml)	**coconut oil for greasing** (optional)	
¼ cup (60 ml)	**nut butter** (almond, cashew, tahini, coconut, etc)	
⅓ cup (75 ml)	**pure maple syrup** (or ½ cup honey)	
2 tsp (10 ml)	**pure vanilla**	
2	**medium ripe bananas, mashed**	
2 cups (500 ml)	**whole grain flour** (whole wheat, kumut, spelt, brown rice)	
4 tsp (20 ml)	**baking powder**	
1 tsp (5 ml)	**ground cinnamon**	
½ tsp (1 ml)	**salt**	
½ cup (25 ml)	**fruit juice or water**	
½ cup (125 ml)	**dried cranberries**	
½ cup (125 ml)	**nuts** (pecans, walnuts, etc)	
¾-1 cup (175-250 ml)	**dark chocolate chips**	

1 batch frosting - see Section 3
- ▸ TOFU MAPLE CAKE ICING
- ▸ CASHEW COCONUT CRÈME
- ▸ CARAMEL FROSTING
- ▸ CHOCOLATE CRÈME FROSTING

Preheat oven to 350°F.

Cream the nut butter, maple syrup and vanilla together in a large bowl. Add the mashed banana and beat together.

Mix the dry ingredients in a separate bowl and then add them to the wet ingredients.

As you blend the batter, drizzle the liquid in small amounts, adding a bit more liquid if necessary.

Fold in fruit, nuts and chocolate chips.

Bake in greased or paper cup lined muffin pans or one loaf pan.

Cupcakes/Muffins: fill pans ¾ full and bake for 25-30 minutes.

Loaf or cake: Bake 55-60 minutes.

Test for doneness with a toothpick or skewer.

Cool completely and frost.

Chocolate: luscious, lumpy, load of love!

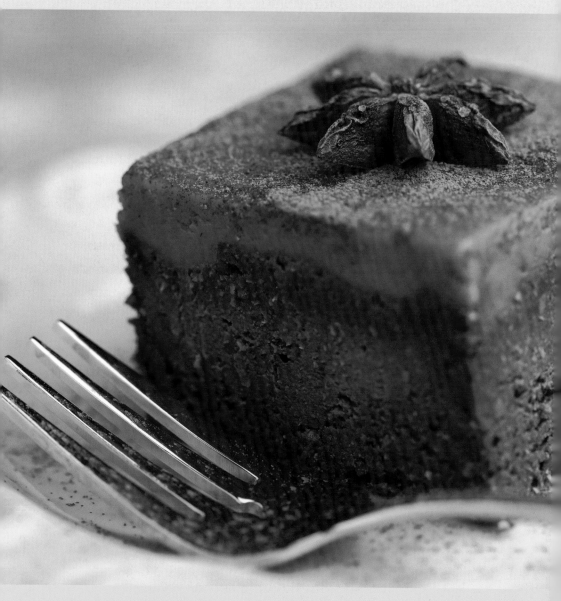

Tester Comments

"Mmmm…spices and molasses in a warm gingerbread…only gets better with the addition of the cocoa."

SPICY CHOCOLATE GINGERBREAD CAKE

If you love a gingerbread cake, you'll love this version…spicy, moist and sweet.

Makes: one 9" cake

1 cup (250 ml)	**nut butter** (tahini, cashew)
½ cup (125 ml)	**blackstrap molasses**
2-3	**ripe bananas, mashed** (approx. 1½ cups 375 ml)
2 cups (500 ml)	**whole grain flour** (wheat, kumut, spelt, oat, brown rice, etc)
2 tsp (10 ml)	**baking powder**
½ cup (60 ml)	**cocoa powder**
1 tsp (5 ml)	**ground ginger powder**
½ tsp (2 ml)	**each: ground cinnamon and nutmeg powder**
⅛ - ¼ tsp (0.5-1 ml)	**cloves** (optional)
⅓ - ½ cup (75-125 ml)	**water**

Preheat oven to 350ºF.

Grease a 9" x 9" square pan.

In a large bowl, cream together the nut butter, molasses and banana using a hand blender or mixer. Add the dry ingredients to the bowl. While mixing batter add the water in splashes until combined. Pour batter into the prepared pan.

Bake for 30-35 minutes until lightly browned and toothpick comes out clean. Cool for 10 minutes in pan then remove and cool on a wire rack.

Serving Suggestions:
Frost with one of the following, if desired - Section 3:

▶ CHOCOLATE CRÈME FROSTING

▶ CARAMEL FROSTING

VARIATION

▶ Serve with applesauce in place of frosting.
▶ Sprinkle ½ cup chocolate chips into batter before baking.

Can you imagine a day when doctor says to patient…"take two squares of chocolate and call me in the morning"?!

DID YOU KNOW?

Orange zest is high in bioflavanoids and calcium. Use certified organically grown oranges to avoid the pesticides on the skin.

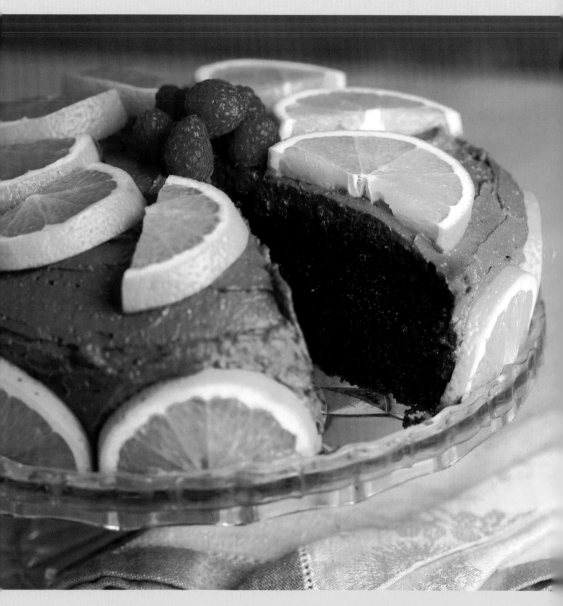

Tester Comments

"Orange and chocolate have an affinity for each other. I'm so impressed with this cake. I can hardly wait to make it again for another occasion."

ORANGE CHOCOLATE CAKE WITH ZESTY CRÈME FROSTING

Light and fluffy and full of flavour, this whole grain cake is my daughter Jacqueline's delicious creation, and is always a hit. It is also lovely decorated or served with fresh berries.

Makes: Two - 8" cakes or one layer cake

3 cups (750 ml)	**whole grain pastry flour**
2 cups (500 ml)	**raw sugar**
½ cup (125 ml)	**cocoa powder**
2 tsp (10 ml)	**baking soda**
½ tsp (2 ml)	**salt**
1 tsp (5 ml)	**ground cinnamon**
2 cups (500 ml)	**orange juice**
½ cup (125 ml)	**olive oil**
2 tsp (15 ml)	**orange zest**
2 tsp (10 ml)	**vanilla**
2 tsp (10 ml)	**vinegar**
½ cup (125 ml)	**raspberry jam**
1 batch	**ZESTY ORANGE CHOCOLATE CRÈME FROSTING - Section 3**
1	**whole orange** (for decorating)

Note:

▸ I use apple cider vinegar.

▸ Whole grain pastry flour is finely ground flour that produces a bit lighter product. If you only have regular whole grain flour, put it through your blender for about 30 seconds.

Preheat oven to 350°F. Grease 2 - 8" pans with coconut or olive oil.

Wash and zest an orange.

In a large bowl, mix together the dry ingredients with a whisk or large spoon.

In a medium bowl, combine wet ingredients.

Pour the wet ingredients into the dry and stir until combined, but do not over mix. Scrape batter into cake pan(s) and bake until a toothpick or skewer comes out clean, approximately 25 - 30 minutes. Cool completely on racks.

LAYERS: Spread raspberry jam or frosting between cooled cake layers (if applicable).

Frost with ZESTY ORANGE CHOCOLATE CRÈME FROSTING and decorate with fresh orange slices and optional mint leaves.

Chocolate makes otherwise normal people melt into strange states of ecstasy.

Mandalas, the circle of life, are a symbol of unity. Creating mandalas from sweets and nut meats is a beautiful way to remember the sweetness in our lives and is a wonderful celebratory treat.

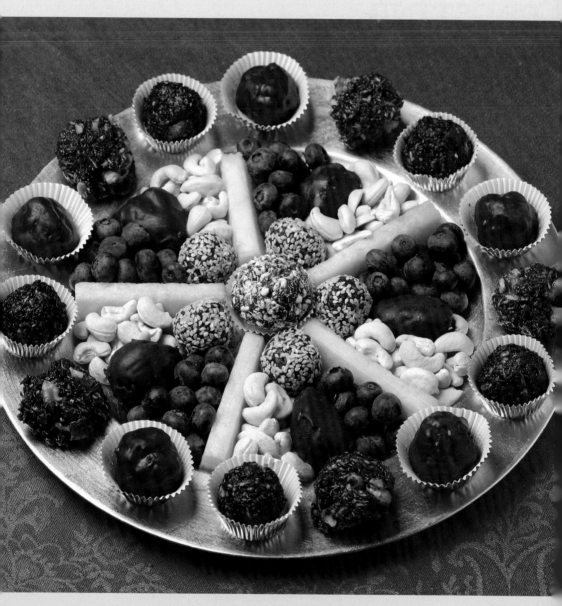

BE CREATIVE AND ENJOY!

CELEBRATION MANDALA

Mandalas are a creative and personal expression. Any variety of colours and textures, however simple or complex, will be brilliant - so don't be afraid to experiment. Each one is unique…so have fun!

Makes: one MANDALA, as large as your plate or tray

Use a variety of the following:

Dried Fruits: **Raisins, cranberries, apricots, dates, prunes, figs, apples, blueberries, mangos, etc.**

Raw or dry roasted Nuts or Seeds: **Almonds, pecans, walnuts, hazelnuts, Brazil nuts, sunflower seeds, pumpkin seeds, etc.**

Fresh Fruit dipped in melted Chocolate: **Strawberries, orange segments, pineapple chunks, etc. See MELTING CHOCOLATE RULES in ABOUT RECIPES section.**

Any of these RECIPES from Section 4:
COCOA MILLET CHEWS
MACADAMIA NUT TRUFFLES
HEALTHY TURTLE BONBONS
TRIPLE OMEGA ENERGY BALLS
SESAME GINGER BLACK BALL BLISS
COCONUT ALMOND JOY BARS

Create this colorful array of fruits and nuts on a large round glass or ceramic plate or tray. Arrange crisscrossing lines for boundaries (eg. sliced apples, oranges, grapes or any of the recipes listed below.)

Fill in the sections with nuts or seeds and dried fruits of various colors and sizes, or any of the different suggested recipes.

Note: Decorative paper candy holders (silver & gold are most attractive) are a great way to display larger items.

Chocolate in the mouth is worth two on the plate.

RECOMMENDED RESOURCES AND REFERENCES

You will find many of the references I used in the following books and for more - see **www.wholefoodsrescue.com**

BOOKS

John Robbins - Book Titles: <u>Diet for a New America; May All Be Fed; Reclaiming our Health; The Awakened Heart; The Food Revolution; Healthy at 100</u>

Sally Errey - <u>Staying Alive! Cookbook for Cancer Free Living; Rooibos Revolution - Recipes for Nature's Healing Tea</u>

Richard Béliveau, Ph.D., Denis Gingras, Ph.D. - <u>Foods That Fight Cancer: Preventing Cancer Through Diet</u>

Carol Off - <u>Bitter Chocolate: Investigating the Dark Side of the World's Most Seductive Sweet</u>

T. Colin Campbell, PhD and Thomas M. Campbell - <u>(The) China Study; Startling Implications for Diet, Weight Loss and Long Term Health</u>

Jane Goodall - <u>Harvest for Hope: A Guide to Mindful Eating</u>

Hale Sofia Schatz - <u>If the Buddha Came to Dinner; How to Nourish Your Body to Awaken Your Spirit</u>

Chloe Doutre-Roussel - <u>The Chocolate Connoisseur; For Everyone with a Passion for Chocolate</u>

<u>Chocolate: The Exquisite Indulgence</u> - Running Room Press

Liz Pearson, R.D. and Mairlyn Smith - <u>Ultimate Foods for Ultimate Health…and don't forget the chocolate!</u>

Cynthia Holzapfel and Laura Holzapfel - <u>Coconut Oil for Health and Beauty</u>

Brenda Davis, RD & Tom Barnard, MD - <u>Defeating Diabetes: A No-Nonsense Approach to Type 2 Diabetes</u>

Brenda Davis, RD & Vesanto Melina, MS, RD - <u>Becoming Vegan: The Complete Guide to Adopting a Healthy Plant-based Diet</u>

B. Davis, Clark, Grogan, Stepaniak - <u>Dairy Free and Delicious</u>

Dr. James D. Krystosik - <u>Carbs from Heaven, Carbs from Hell</u>

Russell Blaylock, MD, Neurosurgeon - <u>Excitotoxins: The Taste that Kills</u>

Richard Rose & Brigitte Mars - <u>HempNut Cookbook</u>

B. Bloomfield, J. Brown, S. Gursche - <u>Flax: The Super Food</u>

Joe Traynor - Honey: The Gourmet Medicine

Robert Cohen - Milk A-Z

Howard F. Lyman - Mad Cowboy

Douglas J. Lisle, PhD & Alan Goldhamer, D.C. - The Pleasure Trap: Mastering the Hidden Force that Undermines Health & Happiness

S. Meyerowitz - Food Combining and Digestion: 101 Ways to Improve Digestion

Rita Elkins - The Complete Fibre Fact Book

Paul Pitchford - Healing with Whole Foods: Oriental Traditions and Modern Nutrition

Dr. Bernard Jensen & Mark Anderson - Empty Harvest: Understanding the Link Between our Food, our Immunity, and our Planet

Annamarie Colbin - Food and Healing

Carolee Bateson-Koch - Allergies: Disease in Disguise

John Matsen, ND - Eating Alive: Prevention Thru Good Digestion

Victoria, Igor, Sergei, and Valya Boutenko - Raw Family: A True Story of Awakening

Sergei and Valya Boutenko - Eating without Heating

Alive Publishing Group - Book Titles: Fats that Heal, Fats that Kill; Hard to Swallow - the truth about Food Additives; Encyclopedia of Natural Healing

WEBSITES

Victoria Laine - **www.wholefoodsrescue.com**

John Robbins - **www.foodrevolution.org www.healthyat100.org**

Chocolate Slavery - **www.foodrevolution.org slavery_chocolate.htm**

What about Soy? - **www.foodrevolution.org what_about_soy.htm**

Physicians Committee for Responsible Medicine - **www.pcrm.org**
Washington, D.C. (Information and on-line bookstore.) -
www.healthyschoollunches.org changes non-dairy.html

Food and Agriculture Organization of the United Nations -
www.fao.org newsroom en news 2006 1000448 index.html

Chocoholic Club - **www.virtualchocoholics** by John Scalzi, called the Unstoppable -
Double-Fudge Chocolate Mudslide Explosion.

Boutenko Family - **www.therawfamily.com**

INDEX

ABOUT THE AUTHOR

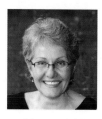

Victoria Laine, N.C.P., is a holistic nutrition counsellor and teacher, yoga instructor, and the mother of two amazing daughters. Victoria received her nutrition education at the Canadian School of Natural Nutrition. She is also a professional member of the International Organization of Nutritional Consultants (IONC). Victoria provides individual and family consulting services, speaks to groups on nutrition and wellness topics, and teaches Whole Food cooking-nutrition classes at the Northern Alberta Institute of Technology (NAIT) in Edmonton, AB. Go to **www.wholefoodsrescue.com** to learn more about the upcoming books she is working on.

INTRODUCTION TO
WHOLEFOODS TO THE
RESCUE! SERIES

Wholefoods to the Rescue! Recipe & Nutrition Guides are being created and published in response to the growing need for nutrition information and recipes that inspire and support even the most beginner cook to prepare basic healthy food and to eat responsibly in today's hectic world.

WHAT ARE WHOLE FOODS?

Whole foods and whole food ingredients:

▸ are as close to their natural state as possible;

▸ have not been highly processed or refined, (like white flour and white sugar have), or altered in ways that significantly decrease their nutritional value;

▸ have not had anything taken away, or added to them (eg. bran and germ removed from grains, or preservatives added) to decrease their quality;

▸ are nutritionally dense and health enhancing;

▸ include whole grains, legumes, vegetables, fruits, nuts and seeds.

There is clear evidence that a simple, whole food, plant based, balanced diet can prevent and sometimes even reverse heart disease and diabetes. It's exciting to see the healing power of food, along with other healthy habits, reverse type 2 diabetes, high cholesterol and triglycerides, high blood pressure, and obesity using this whole foods diet, often within only a matter of months.

UPCOMING TITLES:

▸ **LESS STRESS MEALS IN MINUTES**

▸ **DINNERS-IN-A-DASH**

▸ **LICKETY-SPLIT-LUNCHES**

▸ **BREAKFASTS-IN-A-BLINK**

BOOK ORDER FORM

Online orders: **www.healthbychocolatebook.com**
www.wholefoodsrescue.com

Email orders: **orders@healthbychocolatebook.com**

Postal orders: **OwL Medicine Books, PO Box 79042, 926 Ash Street,**
Sherwood Park, AB T8A 2G1 CANADA

Telephone orders: **(780) 416-4244**

I understand that I may return this book for a full refund - for any reason, no questions asked.

For special offers, bulk ordering discounts (including fundraisers), and International ordering, see website or call (780) 416-4244. Prices are in Canadian dollars and are exclusive of Government Sales Tax. Also see our website or call for a list of our distributors.

Please send the first book of the *Wholefoods to the Rescue!* Series
HEALTH BY CHOCOLATE: radical new recipes & nutrition know-how __$24.95 CDN__

Qty_____ Unit Price_____ Total _____
(to address below)

*Free Shipping
to Canadian addresses.
(Subject to change without notice.)
Please allow a minimum of 4-10 days for delivery. Please call for Rush Orders (charges apply).
Contact us for U.S. Shipping.

Qty_____ Unit Price_____ Total _____
(to other addresses provided)

Sub Total _____

Add Taxes 6% (Sub Total x 0.06) _____

◄······ Add Shipping for Rush and U.S. Orders* _____

Total Paid (CDN) _____

Name:_____ Contact Phone#:_____

Address 1:_____

Address 2:_____

City:_____ Province:_____

Postal/Zip Code:_____ Country:_____

E-mail:_____

MAIL ORDERS: ☐ money order ☐ cheque (make payable to: Wholefoods Rescue)
Note: Your order will be shipped after your cheque clears our bank. Please allow an extra 5 days for shipping.

PAYPAL: Through PayPal we accept Visa, Mastercard, American Express, and Discover. PayPal also accepts cash payments or echeck.

Card Number:_____ Expiry Date:_____ / _____

Name on Card:_____ Signature:_____

UPCOMING TITLES:
☐ Please notify me when the next **Wholefoods to the Rescue!** book is available
(Less Stress Meals in Minutes; Dinners-in-a-Dash, Lickety-Split-Lunches, Breakfasts-in-a-Blink)

ORDER NOW
www.wholefoodsrescue.com
www.healthbychocolatebook.com
(780) 416-4244

HEALTH BY CHOCOLATE

radical new recipes & nutrition know-how

makes an irresistable gift!

We will ship free of charge within Canada, **HEALTH BY CHOCOLATE**
to the recipient(s) of your choice. (Contact us for U.S. shipping).
Provide us with full mailing addresses below. You can also include a greeting or short note.

Mail___copies to:_____
_{Name and full address}
_____
_____

Message to: _____
_{Include up to 3 lines}
_____
_____

Mail___copies to:_____
_{Name and full address}
_____
_____

Message to: _____
_{Include up to 3 lines}
_____
_____

Mail___copies to:_____
_{Name and full address}
_____
_____

Message to: _____
_{Include up to 3 lines}
_____
_____

Mail___copies to:_____
_{Name and full address}
_____
_____

Message to: _____
_{Include up to 3 lines}
_____
_____

Go to **www.healthbychocolatebook.com** or call (780) 416-4244,
for bulk discount rates so you can gift your spouse,
secretaries, co-workers, employees, volunteers, or your friends
with **HEALTH BY CHOCOLATE!**